# OPPORTUNITIES AND OPTIONS IN MEDICAL CAREERS

Ruth Chambers,
Kay Mohanna
and
Steve Field

With contributions from
Muriel Cohen

Foreword by
John Temple

Radcliffe Medical Press Ltd
18 Marcham Road, Abingdon, Oxon OX14 1AA

British Library Cataloguing in Publication Data

A catalogue record for this book is available from the British Library.

ISBN 1 85775 451 4

Typeset by Advance Typesetting Ltd, Oxon.
Printed and bound by TJ International Ltd, Padstow, Cornwall

# ► CONTENTS

## 2 Effective careers guidance and career counselling     21

## 3 Where are you now – career review and assessment     41

## 4 Structured training for medicine     55

# ▶ FOREWORD

The *modern and dependable* National Health Service relies on motivated and highly trained doctors, nurses and other health-care professionals. This workforce needs to be responsive to the rapid pace of change in science and medicine in order to deliver the highest quality care that our patients deserve. We must therefore ensure that not only is the workforce motivated and trained but also able to adapt to the changing environment.

Career planning is essential at all stages of a doctor's career to ensure that the right person is recruited and subsequently retained in the health service and that the individual's own needs are met. It is, however, evident that many students apply for and then enter medical school without informed guidance about the realities of being a doctor and that few doctors have access to impartial career advice, guidance and counselling from informed advisers.[1] There is evidence from many different organizations outside the NHS that the number of people leaving their jobs is reduced by good career guidance.[2]

The authors have many years of experience in careers counselling and in running training courses for those who provide careers advice. This book draws heavily on their experience and fills a gap in the information currently available for all those planning a career in medicine, as well as those already in an established medical career. It gives practical advice for those applying for jobs and provides a valuable source of help for careers advisers and counsellors. It will provide a valuable resource for schools, universities, postgraduate centres and training practice libraries. I commend it to you.

Professor John Temple
Special Adviser to the Chief Medical Officer
Chairman Conference of Postgraduate Medical Deans
*May 2000*

# References

1   Chambers R (1996) *Availability of Career Guidance for General Practice in England and Wales in 1995.* University of Keele, Keele.

2   Killeen J, White M and Watts A (1992) *The Economic Value of Careers Guidance.* Policy Studies Institute, London.

Medical career counselling should be available for all doctors throughout their careers, and not just for students and newly qualified doctors who are unsure of their career direction. In the past, few doctors have been able to access good information and advice about the vast range of options and opportunities. A flat career structure and poor match between doctors' personalities and their career specialties contribute to creating the high levels of stress present in the medical profession. Most established doctors feel that they ended up in their current posts through chance conversations, hearing of opportunities through the grapevine, rather than by considered career planning.

This book was originally devised to help doctors in posts that involve giving careers advice, guidance or counselling to other doctors. This might be in having responsibilities for doctors in training, such as being a GP trainer, GP course organiser, GP tutor, clinical tutor or college tutor; or where jobs such as those of BMA representatives or health authority medical advisers encourage established doctors to approach the post-holders for help with their careers. But it was obvious that many of those giving medical careers advice, guidance or counselling, also want to receive it. And it is only possible to be a good medical career counsellor if you have a well-developed understanding and insight into your own career development. So, the material in this book has evolved to meet the needs of those wanting to gain insight into their own career development, to help them with career planning from their own perspectives, as well as helping medical colleagues with their careers.

Giving medical careers advice, guidance and counselling can be an involved process that requires dedicated time and updating on changes in regulations on training and appointments, to be able to help those with complex problems such as arise from geographical constraints, disabilities, mental health problems, disenchantment and poor performance.

This book should help medical readers to understand the differences between careers advice, guidance and counselling, and what each process entails. It helps medical careers advisers and counsellors with the processes of career counselling: 'What is the current situation?' and 'What would it look like, if it were better?' The case histories of medics in 30 examples of medical career specialties describe what's entailed and inform the third stage in the career counselling process: 'How can this be achieved?'

Ruth Chambers
Kay Mohanna
Steve Field
*May 2000*

**Ruth Chambers** has been a GP for 20 years. Her previous experience has encompassed a wide range of research and educational activities. She is currently the Professor of Primary Care Development at the Centre for Health Policy and Practice at Staffordshire University. She was a GP trainer for four years with challenging GP registrars.

Ruth regards career development as a positive way to minimise the significant stresses in a doctor's life. She has researched into the needs for medical career support services and organised career counselling skills training. One of the most formative experiences of her own career was an in-depth career review with Medical Forum.

**Kay Mohanna** is a GP and lecturer in medical education at Staffordshire University. She has made several changes in her life and career without the benefit of objective advice. She was the Royal College of General Practitioners' Midland Faculty young practitioners' fellow in 1997/8. Her research revealed a need for career support for GPs in the early years of practice and resulted in the publication of a resource booklet. It also led to Kay initiating 'Bridging the Gap', a professional development course.

As joint organiser of four young practitioner conferences she has met many doctors whose experiences illustrate their need for interested careers advisers with objective and up-to-date information about the alternative pathways available within medicine.

**Steve Field** is the Director of Postgraduate GP Education for the West Midlands and sponsored the medical career counselling research and skills training that informed much of the material in this book. Steve is the vice-chair of the Committee of GP Education Directors (COGPED). He has been a GP since 1986 and is a GP principal in inner-city Birmingham. He is a former course organiser for the Worcester Vocational Training Scheme.

# ▶ ACKNOWLEDGEMENTS

We wish to thank Muriel Cohen, career consultant, for her contribution to Chapters 1 and 2. She has enhanced our understanding of careers development and the potential of career counselling through her friendship and the medical career counselling skills training workshops she has facilitated. We also wish to thank the doctors who have contributed their past medical histories and described the symptoms and signs of their current careers in our case studies.

# ABBREVIATIONS

| | |
|---|---|
| A&E | Accident and Emergency |
| CCST | certificate of completion of specialist training |
| CME | continuing medical education |
| COGPED | Committee of GP Education Directors |
| COPMeD | Committee of Postgraduate Medical Deans |
| CPD | continuing professional development |
| DPGPE | Dean/Director of Postgraduate GP Education |
| EEA | European Economic Area |
| FRCAnaes | Fellow of the Royal College of Anaesthetists |
| FRCR | Fellow of the Royal College of Radiologists |
| FRCS | Fellow of the Royal College of Surgeons |
| FTTA | fixed-term training appointment |
| GMC | General Medical Council |
| GMS | General Medical Services (those services provided by general practitioners) |
| GUM | Genito-urinary medicine |
| IELTS | International English Language Testing System |
| JCPTGP | Joint Committee on Postgraduate Training for General Practice |
| LAS | locum appointment, service |
| LAT | locum appointment, training |
| LMC | local medical committee |
| MADEL | medical and dental education levy |
| MBA | Masters in Business Administration |
| MFPHM | Member of the Faculty of Public Health Medicine |
| MRCGP | Member of the Royal College of General Practitioners |
| MRCP | Member of the Royal College of Physicians |
| NICE | National Institute for Clinical Excellence |
| NMET | Non-Medical Education and Training (consortium) |

| | |
|---|---|
| NSF | National Service Framework |
| NTN | national training number |
| ODTS | Overseas Doctors Training Scheme |
| PCG | primary care group |
| PCT | primary care trust |
| PLAB | Professional and Linguistic Assessment Board |
| PMS | personal medical services (pilot) |
| PRHO | pre-registration house officer |
| RCGP | Royal College of General Practitioners |
| RCN | Royal College of Nursing |
| SHO | senior house officer |
| SpR | specialist registrar |
| STA | specialist training authority |
| TWES | training and work experience scheme |
| UKReA | United Kingdom Conference of Regional Advisers |
| VTN | visiting training number |
| VTS | vocational training scheme |

# GLOSSARY OF TERMS

- **Career counselling**: is an umbrella term for the process of enabling somebody to evaluate their current career and identify what steps are needed in order to change. It will usually include identification of a person's strengths and weaknesses in relation to work options and may also include careers information.
- **Careers guidance**: this is personal and directive, and provides *advice* within the context of the career opportunities that are available.
- **Careers information**: covers the facts about the qualifications and experience needed for alternative career pathways and the opportunities that there are for career progression; that is, the number and type of posts available at a particular level and in a particular specialty and details of the qualifications and training necessary.
- **Clinical governance**: a system being implemented throughout the NHS which will assure the public of minimum standards, and encourage good practice and the delivery of cost-effective care by the NHS workforce as a whole.
- **Co-mentoring**: (see 'mentoring') where the process of mentoring is 'non-hierarchical, involving the co-mentees helping and supporting each other in learning'.[1]
- **Coaching**: the process of motivating, encouraging and helping an individual to improve their skills, knowledge and attitudes in a framework of goal setting and achievement.
- **Continuing professional development**: 'a process of lifelong learning for all individuals and teams which enables professionals to expand and fulfil their potential and which also meets the needs of patients and delivers the health and health care priorities of the NHS'.[1]
- **Mentor**: an experienced, highly regarded, empathetic person who guides another individual in the development of

his or her reflection, learning and personal, professional and career development.

► **Mentoring**: 'an ancient process of learning facilitation by mutual professional support, traditionally given by a senior to a junior colleague'.[1]

► **Peer appraisal**: the process by which colleagues identify and constructively discuss each other's strengths, weaknesses and learning needs within a supportive environment.

► **Personal learning plan**: a document describing an individual's learning objectives, the processes by which these objectives are defined and expected to be achieved, and how the achievement of these objectives will be evaluated.

► **Portfolio**: a collection of evidence demonstrating how personal learning has been fulfilled.

► **Reflection**: the process whereby people actively deliberate on their performance or the care they deliver and identify their strengths and weaknesses (as individuals or in groups).

► **Revalidation**: a compulsory episodic affirmation that a doctor continues to be fit to practise.

► **Training**: a process which is planned to facilitate learning so that people can become effective in carrying out aspects of their work.

► **Training needs analysis**: includes the three stages of identifying the range and extent of training needs in relation to the learner, the patient and the health service; specifying those needs precisely; analysing how best those needs might be met.

## Reference

1    Chief Medical Officer (1998) *A Review of Continuing Professional Development in General Practice*. Department of Health, London.

# CHAPTER 1

# Introduction to career planning for doctors

Career planning is a must at all stages of a medical career, for medical students or young doctors uncertain of their career paths, for established doctors faced with a range of career opportunities and dilemmas, or when thinking of retirement.[1] A career review should consider:

- *Who you are and where you are now.*
- *How satisfied you are with your career and life.*
- *Whether you are ready to make a change.*

and plan:

- *Where you want to be.*
- *How you are going to get there.*
- *What you will do if you do not get there.*

Your career plans may centre on developing your particular skills and interests within the specialty in which you are working so that you function more effectively. You may want to develop your career so that you become more specialised in a particular clinical or managerial area. You might want more variety in your work and decide to develop a parallel area of interest or a new skill that enhances your current post. It may be promotion that you are after with more status or responsibility. You may crave for a complete change; in a new career that is a natural extension of your current work, or as a fresh start in a different career within or outside medicine.

---

**Career life planning includes:**[2]

- ▶ identifying relevant experience, personal resources and skills
- ▶ clarifying hopes and ambitions for development
- ▶ describing potential barriers to achievement
- ▶ identifying career options.

---

Most doctors report that they have never received any careers guidance or counselling. They applied for posts as opportunities cropped up with little forward planning. The sort of careers guidance described by the minority of doctors who have received careers help in the past, has been the 'Be like me' kind, with senior doctors describing their own careers as role models to be followed. All doctors in training should have access to regular careers advice and review. But a national survey of the extent of careers guidance and advice available found that services were patchy, with few junior doctors, GP registrars and established doctors having access to well-informed, impartial careers advisers.[3] The British Medical Association (BMA) advocates the setting up of medical careers services that are: 'available, accessible, appropriate, accurate, impartial, confidential, performed by people who have been trained to do it, and responsive to culture and gender'.[4]

---

**Doctors' experiences of receiving (or not) careers advice**

In one study capturing doctors' previous experience of careers advice or guidance, 17 of the 36 doctors interviewed could not recall ever having received any kind of careers advice or guidance at school, before, during or since medical training.[5] Of the 19 doctors who reported receiving any kind of careers advice or guidance, all but three described it as 'informal' or 'ad hoc'. The majority

*continued*

said that the careers advice received had been about the particular specialty in which they were training, rather than encouraging them to consider a range of career options.

Most who had received advice, had sought people out themselves for an informal chat about a particular career specialty. Several had received unsolicited negative advice warning them off particular specialties, for example: 'the professor of surgery in my house job said "I don't think you are cut out to be a surgeon – have you thought of paediatrics?"' Several now regretted being influenced by such off-putting advice. Only one of the six doctors who had made a major career change in the past had received formal career counselling. The three doctors who reported receiving formal career counselling had consulted advisers who, as far as they knew were not trained to provide career counselling.

There are gender differences in choice of specialty, likelihood of progressing to senior positions and proportions who work less than full time. Men are more likely to choose their specialties based on 'interest in the specialty', 'promotion' and 'financial prospects'. Women more often choose 'close contact with patients', 'a job in the right geographical area', 'fit in with family life' and 'availability of part-time work' as important features of their selected career specialties.[6]

## Factors to consider in *choosing* a career specialty or interest[1,7]

When reviewing your current job or weighing up the potential for a career move, you should consider the match between you and the job as to whether:

► you have the sort of personality that fits with the requirements of the job
► you have the appropriate skills, training and experience

▶ you have sufficient job satisfaction and interest in your work
▶ you are sufficiently motivated to work effectively
▶ the job fits with your ethics, inner values and boundaries
▶ the job provides the balance you want between work and your off-duty life.

Reflect on what you are looking for from your work:

▶ the kind of work you enjoy – routine, exciting, prestigious, quiet and steady
▶ the setting in which you want to work – community, hospital, rural, urban, travel
▶ the type of people for whom you want to care – the ages and characteristics of patients
▶ the type of people with whom you want to work and whether in a small team or big organisation
▶ the extent of patient contact that suits you
▶ the level of income you consider (i) essential and (ii) desirable
▶ the working hours, holidays, study leave: how the hours fit with your current state and future domestic plans
▶ opportunities for parallel career interests such as research, writing, education, consultancy, private work or work-related hobbies
▶ the extent of professional autonomy and responsibility you want.

You will also need to take account of:

▶ the details of any training required – hours, practical difficulties, examinations
▶ the job prospects of alternative career paths: the opportunities for you to progress.

## Job satisfaction and career fulfilment

Job satisfaction is known to protect doctors from the effects of stress from work; so increasing your job satisfaction is one of the best ways to 'stress-proof' yourself against the pressures and demands of a job.[1,8,9] You will minimise the effects of the elements of the job you find more stressful if you enjoy your job, feel valued and are in control of your everyday work. Low job satisfaction can affect performance – one example is the link between low job satisfaction and poor prescribing practice.

Female doctors are more satisfied with their hours of work and rates of pay than male colleagues, whereas male GPs find managing and organising practice work more rewarding than women do. Studies of GPs' job satisfaction have shown a downward trend since the late 1980s, with satisfaction gained from the amount of responsibility, variety in the job, physical conditions at work, amount of freedom to choose their own working methods and the recognition they receive for good work. The least satisfied GPs seem to be in the 35 to 44 years age group.[8,10]

# Personality and its effect on work – implications for career choice

Some knowledge of personality is necessary if people are to be helped to realise their potential. The shy, inward-looking person is not going to enjoy a work situation that calls for constant interaction, and the gregarious extrovert will become depressed if deprived of social contact. Understanding your own personal preferences and nature should help you to develop an appropriate career path. Understanding more about what makes another person 'tick' will help you to counsel other people about their career choices. All too often a doctor has spent years notching up exam successes while paying scant attention to what he or she really wants out of life.

Introverted personalities have a tendency to suffer from the effects of stress by the time they have reached their mid-thirties and been working as doctors for ten years; awareness of personality factors may help to match an individual with a career specialty. Doctors who scored more highly on screening tools for psychological symptoms as students are more likely to opt for general practice, psychiatry and anaesthetics. So sensitive people tend to opt for specialties with the closest contact with people.[6]

---

**About personality type**

▶ there is no right or wrong, better or worse combinations of personality types
▶ if you know more about your type you can understand yourself better
▶ each person is unique
▶ everyone uses each of their preferences to some degree
▶ the human personality is too complex for type to explain everything about you.

---

One of the best ways of understanding personality in a short time is to take a validated test such as the Myers Briggs,[11] which measures four bipolar dimensions of personality relating to how people take in information and make decisions. It is thought to be particularly suitable for career development and team building. Another commonly used measure of a personality profile is the 16PF questionnaire, which assesses 16 personality factors. Such tests attempt to show individuals their preferred style of behaviour, in order that they can then choose the aspect of their profession that best matches the way they behave. Failing this, a career counsellor would need to spend much time discussing how someone responds in many situations in order to identify what must ideally be avoided and sought out.

In one 'Return to General Practice' course for GP non-principals, most of the participants rated the workshop session where they received feedback on their Myers Briggs scores as being one of the best of the year's course. Many thought that understanding themselves better would help them find practices where they were more likely to be compatible with the GP partners and practice.

**Take John X for example**

He came for career counselling because he felt that the people with whom he worked disheartened him to such an extent that he could not continue as a GP partner in the practice. When he took a personality test, it revealed that he held an idealistic notion of service which could not be upheld in his very busy urban GP practice. He was an 'ideas' person and most of the things he suggested in the practice were immediately squashed. Rather than giving up the work that he loved, he and the career counsellor discussed his seeking another partnership in a totally different environment, which he has since done. Instead of dreading going to work each day, his enthusiasm has returned and his patients are getting the best service he can deliver.

Opinions about the benefits of psychometric testing are divided. Enthusiasts feel that all those applying for places in medical schools should take personality tests. This would give medical schools additional information about the applicants but would not replace traditional methods of selection. Studies of medical students are in progress to see 'if those who initially described themselves as extroverts may perform better in later clinical stages than those who described themselves as hard-working or conscientious'.[12] The 16PF questionnaire has been used to select medical students in Malaysia, where candidates who were more reserved, less emotionally stable and more apprehensive were found to be more likely to have problems in medical school.[13] The California psychological inventory of 22 personality traits has been used for selecting and studying medical students in Australia and America;[13] American students scored highly for 'achievement via independence' and low for 'self-control', 'desire to create a good impression on others' and 'amicability', although all three low scores were still higher than the average scores of the general population.

Some of the arguments against adopting personality profile testing in the selection of doctors into medicine and for established posts include doubts about the validity of a test. In reality, most established tests include questions that cross-check consistency of response, so that any attempts to give a 'correct' answer should show up in the results. In particular, personality tests such as the Myers Briggs have no 'right' answers. The aim of the test is to identify a person's preferred way of behaving, based on their individual ways of perceiving the world and exercising judgement, in order to help in every aspect of life, career and personal relationships. The idea of selecting a personality type for a particular specialty is flawed, as the resulting team might get on well together but their similarity and lack of diversity may make them less likely to find ways of adapting to change.

## Appreciating your personal ethics and work values

Your ethics set the boundaries as to how far you are prepared to go to get what you want. If you find your personal ethics are not compatible with the job you do, you may find it necessary to leave that specialty or resign from that post. On the other hand, you might feel that you can maintain your standards and integrity despite your environment.[14]

Work values are personal to you too. You will be happiest and most fulfilled in a job that incorporates your main work values. Eight career anchor categories have been identified by Schein[15] to increase people's insights into their strengths and motivation as part of career development: these are technical or functional competence, general managerial competence, autonomy or independence, security or stability, entrepreneurial creativity, service or dedication to a cause, pure challenge, lifestyle. People define their self-image in terms of these traits and come to understand more about their talents, motives and values

– and which of these they would not give up if forced to make a choice.

# Motivation

People are motivated by different things. Money, fame and power are all key motivators. Pride, lust, anger, gluttony, envy, sloth and covetousness are all listed as prime motivators – hopefully not all of these are relevant to any great extent in the NHS! Some of the best motivators for fulfilling doctors' needs[1] are:

- interesting and/or useful work
- sense of achievement
- responsibility
- opportunities for career progression or professional development
- gaining new skills or competencies
- sense of belonging to a Directorate or practice team or the NHS.

Maslow's hierarchy[16] of a person's needs describes how self-esteem and fulfilment are not possible if the basic structure and safety components of their life are insecure. Self-esteem, status and recognition from others are only possible if they are built upon a good social base that includes love, friendship, belonging to groups (work, home, leisure, professional) and social activities. Fulfilment, maturity and wisdom are only possible where all the other conditions encourage growth, personal development and accomplishment. Those in senior positions in the NHS have a responsibility to create a good working environment that motivates staff to perform well.

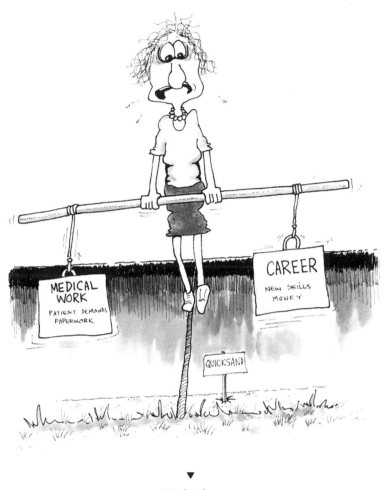

▼
**Motivation**

## Where to work: inner city or rural setting; district general or teaching hospital?

When it comes to settling down in a GP or consultant post you need to consider the location carefully to avoid getting itchy feet soon after you take up your post. You may have little choice because your particular specialty is oversubscribed, or a GP partnership in a leafy suburb is harder to find than an inner-city practice or rural practice without an out-of-hours GP co-operative service.

The following boxes show the features you might want to consider in making your choices.

---

**Factors to consider in opting for a district general hospital or teaching hospital:**[17]

- an academic career or being a generalist – access to university centres
- having a research interest or just doing audit – availability of infrastructure and practical support
- opportunities for teaching
- city preference or rural interests
- family preferences or hobbies
- proximity, access and commitment to relatives
- likely potential for private practice
- availability of junior staff, cover by colleagues, locums
- extent of on-call commitment
- loss of colleagues, sponsors and friends if transfer to other region.

---

**Factors to consider when choosing between inner-city and rural general practice:**[18]

- rural practices tend to be small and remote
- financial insecurity if practice business is dependent on dispensing
- rural practice dispensing profits and payments may make up for the effects of small practice size on income
- the availability of the Associate Practitioner Scheme – deployment of an extra doctor between two single-handed remote practices
- inner-city practices tend to have pockets of deprivation in their patient populations
- continuing education opportunities plentiful in inner cities compared to rural areas
- more opportunities for doctor's family in city locations
- out-of-hours cover may be difficult or non-existent in rural practices
- personal safety may be more of a concern in an inner-city location.

# Getting a sensible balance between work and home lives

There are no hard and fast rules about how much time you should spend on work-related activities compared to the rest of your life. The Health Education Authority's advice to divide your day as:

- ▶ 45–55% on personal needs (including sleeping, chores, basic care)
- ▶ 25–30% on work
- ▶ 20–25% on leisure

makes most doctors who work full time laugh heartily. Only you and your partner at home know if you are getting the balance right. And if you have not got a 'partner at home' to discuss the balance with, maybe it's time you reduced your wholesale commitment to work and socialised more. It is well accepted that if you increase the proportion of work, it is the leisure component that is reduced proportionately.[1]

Developing your career invariably means additional time being spent on preparing for the new stage or change, in pursuit of further qualifications, absorbing extra committee work, looking at the post under consideration, reading around the topic or seeking career counselling. Somehow that additional developmental work has to be fitted into your already-busy life. Don't just add it on top of everything else, but make a concerted effort to stop doing something in its place – delegate chores by employing help, resign from an inessential committee, or whatever is possible.

Part of a career review or career counselling is to give you a chance to work out when is a good time for you to develop your career. You will maybe need to take things more slowly than you would ideally like, to make sure that the work component of your life is manageable and you don't take on so much that you become overstretched, resulting in you becoming ineffective all round.

# The relationship between continuing professional development and careers development

Continuing personal and professional development are integral to maintaining job satisfaction and professional fulfilment. Job satisfaction can be promoted through continuing professional education and development, and opportunities for career advancement.

Every doctor should set out a personal educational development plan that they review each year. Career development should be an integral part of such a plan setting out goals for the forthcoming year and beyond, and realistic ways of achieving those goals. A performance appraisal is a good way to start the plan – as a review of your post by a trusted colleague or mentor, or by a self-assessment.[19]

You cannot consider your own individual needs and plans in isolation from those of the rest of your work team or organisation, or the needs of the NHS as a whole.[19] There needs to be an opening for such a post or the new skills you intend to develop. Figure 1.1 depicts the influences that the priorities and service development needs of a trust or general practice, and the rest of the NHS, have on an individual doctor's own personal, professional and career development. A successful personal development plan must balance these competing influences and pressures while enabling individual doctors to *stay in control* of the development of their careers and working lives and retain their organisation's and colleagues' support.

# The relationship between careers development and workforce planning

Improved and extended medical career counselling services could underpin workforce planning by informing doctors about specialties with more openings and opportunities, and where there are currently unfilled vacancies.

Numbers of GPs rose from 27 420 in 1988 to 29 697 in 1998, an increase of more than 8%, which in real terms has meant an increased ratio of 55.4 GPs per 100 000 population in 1998 compared with 53.2 GPs to 100 000 population in 1988.[20]

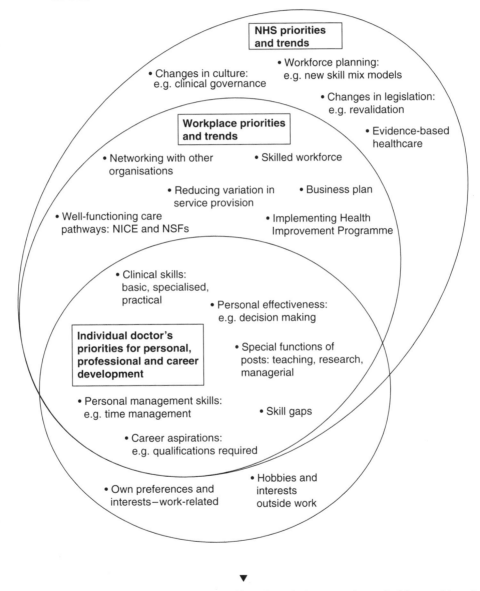

**Figure 1.1: Influences and pressures of NHS and workplace service priorities and trends on an individual doctor's own plan for personal, professional and career development**

The growth in numbers of hospital consultants at an average annual rate of 4% in the last decade has exceeded the 3% average annual growth in numbers of junior doctors. In 1998, 34% of hospital doctors were consultants and 48% were junior doctors. The junior doctor-to-consultant ratio fell from 1.55 to 1 in 1988, to 1.42 to 1 in 1998. Consultants' roles and responsibilities have changed with comparatively fewer junior doctors. Staff-grade posts have almost trebled in five years from just over 1000 in 1993 to nearly 3000 in 1998.[20]

General practitioner registrar numbers dropped by 14% from 1685 in 1988, to 1446 in 1998; although there was an 8% increase in the 1997–98 year compared to the numbers in the previous 12 months. Partnership sizes varied over the 1988–98 decade; numbers of single-handed GPs fell by 8%, and the numbers of GPs in partnerships of six or more doctors rose by 54%; the numbers of GPs in partnerships of three or fewer fell by 9%.[20]

The majority of hospital consultants (85% of male and 71% of female consultants) hold full- or maximum part-time contracts. An even higher proportion of junior doctors have full-time posts (96% of males and 90% of females). The majority of GPs continue to work full time to provide at least 26 hours of patient contact time; 5% worked less than full time in 1988 compared with 16% in 1998. Almost two-fifths (39%) of women GPs worked less than full time in 1998.[20]

A third of hospital medical staff are women; numbers have increased by 72% since 1988. But the proportion of women in senior positions has grown more slowly, with 14% of consultants being women in 1988 compared with 21% in 1998. The number of overseas trained doctors who qualified outside the European Economic Area (EEA) who are working in the NHS increased from 23% in 1993, to 25% in 1998; two-thirds of these doctors are employed as junior doctors and most hold staff and associate specialist posts. Numbers of doctors working in the NHS who qualified outside the UK but inside the EEA also rose from 5 to 6% over the same period.[20]

The tables below give the official statistics for the numbers of doctors employed in England in 1998. There have been increases in the numbers of consultants in all the main specialties, with the most marked rises being in paediatrics and accident and emergency work.

**Table 1.1: Numbers of doctors by specialty group working for the NHS (in England)[20]**

|  | 1988 | 1998 |
|---|---|---|
| All hospital medical staff | 37 600 | 54 420 |
| Public health medical staff | 670 | 820 |
| Community medical staff | 2120 | 1040 |
| All GPs | 25 322 | 27 392 |

**Table 1.2: Numbers of doctors by grade working for the NHS (in England)[20]**

|  | 1993 | 1998 |
|---|---|---|
| *Hospital based* |  |  |
| Hospital consultant | 15 210 | 19 380 |
| Associate specialist | 840 | 1220 |
| Staff grade | 1050 | 2870 |
| Hospital registrar* | 9750 | 11 060 |
| Senior house officer | 11 880 | 14 600 |
| House officer | 3080 | 3440 |
| Hospital practitioner | 160 | 180 |
| Clinical assistant | 1830 | 1640 |
| *General practitioners* |  |  |
| Unrestricted principals / PMS GPs | 26 289 | 27 392 |
| Restricted principals | 147 | 97 |
| Assistants | 495 | 701 |
| GP registrars | 1529 | 1446 |
| Salaried doctors and PMS employed |  | 61 |

* Specialist registrar grade introduced in 1996.

**Table 1.3: Numbers of hospital medical consultants by specialty group (in England)[20]**

|                              | 1988 | 1998 |
|------------------------------|------|------|
| General medicine             | 3160 | 4810 |
| Paediatrics                  | 660  | 1300 |
| Accident and emergency       | 180  | 420  |
| Surgical group               | 2970 | 4190 |
| Obstetrics and gynaecology   | 750  | 1040 |
| Anaesthetics                 | 1970 | 2960 |
| Radiology                    | 1050 | 1510 |
| Clinical oncology            | 210  | 300  |
| Pathology group              | 1480 | 1890 |
| Psychiatry group             | 1900 | 2630 |

The 1000 new undergraduate training places for medical students in England from year 2000 onwards will increase the annual intake of UK medical schools by nearly 20%. The number of GPs employed through personal medical services pilot schemes has risen since 170 new approvals in 1999.[20]

## Career tracks of young doctors

The BMA is tracking a cohort of 509 doctors who graduated from UK medical schools in 1995. Four years on, 70% have a strong desire to practise medicine, 25% have a lukewarm desire, 3% a weak desire and 3% regret becoming doctors. Two-thirds intend to be hospital doctors, 25% to enter general practice and 6% are still unsure. The majority of those opting for general practice are women (70%); the majority of those choosing surgery are men (80%). Since graduation 1% had left medicine as a career and another 1% are working as doctors overseas and do not intend to return to work in the UK. One in five of the cohort had spent some time out of the workforce in the previous year, usually working overseas or travelling abroad. Two-thirds of the women and one-quarter of the men were considering flexible training in the future.[21]

# References

1 Chambers R (1999) *Survival Skills for GPs*. Radcliffe Medical Press, Oxford.

2 Dainow S (1998) *Working and Surviving in Organisations*. Wiley, Chichester.

3 Chambers R (1996) *Careers in general practice – towards a more informed choice. Availability of career guidance for general practice in England and Wales in 1995*. A Royal College of General Practitioners' Revaluing General Practice Initiative. Keele University, Stoke-on-Trent.

4 British Medical Association (1996) *Guidelines for the Provision of Careers Services for Doctors*. British Medical Association, London.

5 Chambers R (1998) Careers counselling for general practice. *West Midlands J Primary Care*. **4**: 32–9.

6 Baldwin P (1999) Cohort studies of Scottish medical school graduates. In *1st Oxford Conference on Medical Careers*. Oxford University, Oxford.

7 Bache J (1999) Choosing a career. *BMJ Classified, Career Focus*. **8 May**: 2–3.

8 Sutherland V and Cooper C (1993) Identifying distress among general practitioners: predictors of psychological ill-health and job dissatisfaction. *Soc Sci Med*. **37**(5): 575–81.

9 Ramirez A, Graham J, Richards M *et al.* (1996) Mental health of hospital consultants: the effects of stress and satisfaction at work. *Lancet*. **347**: 724–8.

10 Sutherland V and Cooper C (1992) Job stress, satisfaction, and mental health among general practitioners before and after introduction of new contract. *BMJ*. **304**: 1545–8.

11 Myers I and Myers P (1995) *Gifts Differing. Understanding personality type*. Davies-Black, California.

12 Wojtas O and Currie J (1999) Psychometric testing could cut student doctor drop-outs. *The Times Higher*. **8 January**: 6.

13 Cook M (1998) New approaches to selecting medical staff. *BMJ Classified, Career Focus*. **14 March**: 2–3.

14 NHS Executive (1994) *Career Management Programme for Women*. Domino Consultancy, Leicestershire.

15 Schein E (1996) *Career Anchors: discovering your real values*. Pfeiffer, Oxford.

16 Maslow AH (1970) *Motivation and Personality*. Harper & Row, New York.

17 Sellar W (1999) District general hospital or teaching hospital? *BMJ Classified, Career Focus*. **20 February**: 2–3.

18 Royal College of General Practitioners (1999) Rural general practice. *RCGP Information Sheet No 23*. Royal College of General Practitioners, London.

19 Chambers R and Wall D (1999) *Teaching Made Easy: a manual for health professionals*. Radcliffe Medical Press, Oxford.

20 Davies J (ed) (1999) *Employing medical and dental staff. The monthly report on employment trends and data*. Chamberlain Dunn, Gothic House, Richmond.

21 British Medical Association (1999) *Fourth Report – March 1999*. Workforce participation and career intentions three years after graduation. Health Policy and Economic Research Unit, British Medical Association, London.

# CHAPTER 2

# Effective careers guidance and career counselling

Without adequate medical career support services doctors may remain ignorant of the options available, spend too much time in posts that are not ultimately relevant and even be lost to the profession altogether if they do not find their right niche.

*Careers information* gives the facts about the qualifications and experience needed for alternative career pathways and the opportunities that there are for career progression. This includes written and/or verbal information about the number and type of posts available at various levels in particular specialties and details of the qualifications and training necessary.[1]

*Careers guidance* is more personal and directive, and provides *advice* within the context of the opportunities that are available. It is useful for those who have not made a career decision or are unaware of the best way of achieving their career goals.[1]

## What is career counselling?

*Career counselling* is an intensive process requiring specialist skills. Career counselling is an umbrella term for the process of enabling somebody to evaluate their current situation and identify what steps are needed in order to change. It will usually include identification of a person's strengths and weaknesses in relation to work options and possibly careers information. The extent and type of help and support doctors need depends on their personal circumstances; *career counselling* may be more appropriate than *careers guidance*. Career counselling has the potential to help doctors at all stages of their careers but may be particularly important for non-principals thinking of returning to general practice, young doctors who want to discuss flexible career paths rather than long-term commitments and for the one-third of pre-registration doctors who do not end up in their first choice of career.

Career counselling is a *process* and not an *event*. It involves being alongside someone, listening to them carefully and supporting them as they work through their problems. This process should enable people to recognise and utilise their own resources to manage career-related problems and make career-related decisions.

In most respects, career counselling is similar to any other kind of counselling in that it offers a framework for looking at problem situations and provides support to enable the person with the problem situation to undertake whatever changes they may decide to make. People come to career counselling for all sorts of reasons. Within the medical profession doctors may feel that they are not advancing as they should do. They may feel trapped in work that no longer challenges or satisfies them. They may feel that the work environment and the team with whom they work are not giving them the support they need. They may feel so alienated that their performance falls below acceptable standards. Whatever the reason, successful career counselling will enable that person to identify the issues that need to be dealt with and mobilise the resources they need to improve matters.

The use of the word *counselling* embodies an *attitude* that anyone who counsels another must attempt to provide. That attitude is summed up by Carl Rogers, an influential figure in the world of counselling, who said that three things are needed:[2]

- respect
- a non-judgemental attitude
- honesty in dealing with the other person.

Equipped with these attributes, an informed medical career counsellor can help colleagues to work out solutions to their difficulties as part of the career counselling process.

The kind of thinking patterns from which doctors might benefit from talking things through with a career counsellor who is independent, well-informed and non-judgemental are when:

- they are not solving problems which they have the resources to solve
- their thinking is clouded
- they are putting off making necessary decisions
- they seem unaware of the consequences of their behaviour
- they are engaging in self-defeating behaviour
- they are not mobilising their energies
- they are not responding to the usual motivators
- they are unaware of their talents and strengths.

## Process

The necessary ingredients for good career counselling are:

- self-knowledge on the part of the 'client'
- awareness of strengths and those areas that are under-developed
- a model from which to work, such as Egan's problem management model[3]
- access to a wide database of job options in the relevant field of work.

The best career counselling takes place when the counsellor and the 'client' engage in a joint exploration of possibilities and generate a range of options for further consideration. It is the overall attitude of the counsellor that can be most beneficial in the helping situation.

# Is providing career counselling for you?

If you are now wondering whether you might become a medical career counsellor, try the following experiment. Consider the list below and try to identify the two categories in which you feel least skilled at present. Then consider the two categories that you currently feel most skilled in using. Consider the implications of this and think of ways of remedying any skill deficits:

▶ giving advice – offering suggestions
▶ offering information
▶ challenging what is said to you
▶ helping another person to express emotion
▶ drawing another person out
▶ encouraging and supporting the other person.

Next make a list of the qualities for which you would look in anyone to whom you felt able to turn for help. Which are the ones that you consider absolutely *essential* and which are the ones that are *desirable*? Reflect on this and start to work out how to acquire these qualities. You will then have embarked on training in career counselling and begun a valuable piece of personal development.

## The difference between hearing and listening

The quality of attention that you bring to the session is achieved by a concentrated form of listening. There is a great deal of difference between *hearing* and *listening*. Hearing is a passive activity while listening is active and requires you to *show* that you have been listening. There is a real difference between the listening which takes place with a patient when taking a case history, and the kind of listening you will need when helping a colleague to reflect on their situation. When taking a case history you are assessing what they say with a view to making a diagnosis. The first step with a colleague is to enable them to express themselves fully and feel understood. This process consists of reflecting back what has been said, paraphrasing and summarising at frequent intervals. Only when someone feels certain that they are understood will they proceed to share their thoughts and feelings.

Remember that the outcome of career counselling should be *action*. People come for counselling because they seek change and most people have the utmost difficulty changing aspects of their thinking and their lives. So the career counsellor needs the ability to see things from the other's point of view and the sensitivity to encourage whatever change is needed.

The three-stage model of problem management of Gerard Egan[3] is particularly useful for career counselling. Essentially it poses the following questions:

1  What is the current situation?
2  What would it look like, if it were better?
3  How can this be achieved?

Using this framework allows the person to tell their story, then to start thinking about what would need to be in place for the situation to be improved and finally to work out an action plan to deliver those changes. Any successful action plan needs a timescale. Discuss what is possible in the short, medium and long term.

# The three-stage model of career counselling

## Stage one

Getting the person to tell their story. Whether this is an easy task or a difficult one will depend to a large degree on the rapport established at the outset, which is why people beginning to use career counselling skills spend a great deal of time communicating their empathy and respect for the other person.

## *Stage two*

Developing a better scenario. Egan[3] suggested that one of the main reasons for the need for career counselling is that the person cannot envisage an improved situation. If the current state of affairs is problematic and unacceptable, help is needed to imagine what might be better. If, for example, a difficulty crops up regarding relationships with other work colleagues, one of the ways in which the situation could be improved would be to devise a strategy to deal with this.

## *Stage three*

Moving towards the preferred scenario. Because many of the people seeking help will hold a blinkered view of what is possible, it is here that many will require most help. Brainstorming throws up many ideas without screening them and is very useful at this stage. Following ideas through to their logical conclusions will enable the person to see what will be the result of each line of action. In this way, many more options are opened up.

# Conducting a career counselling session

Before you start you need to ensure that the conditions in which you will operate are the best you can achieve. Arrange to meet at a specified time without interruptions. Ideally, you need comfortable seating and a relaxed setting. The issues you will want to explore are usually of a sensitive nature, and the more you can put the other person at ease, the better the interaction will be. Setting the boundaries in this way allows the other person to feel that they have your full attention for the stated time.

You must reassure colleagues being counselled that confidentiality is guaranteed, except on certain specific occasions when you may be obliged to set confidentiality aside, such as if the person you are helping has been or is involved in some illegal activity, or patient safety is threatened and the doctor concerned refuses to desist from practising.

Adopt relaxed and positive body language as a career counsellor. Get the person being counselled to start talking about their circumstances; if their problems are overwhelming get them to choose an issue on which to concentrate.

You should allow at least 50 minutes for the session. If the problem is relatively simple, such as helping someone to talk through a choice of options that are all viable in themselves, then one session may be sufficient. But if the person being counselled has a complex problem with potentially serious consequences if he or she takes certain paths, then three or four career counselling sessions may be required.

One of a career counsellor's most productive techniques is to challenge the other person's restrictive attitudes, beliefs or behaviour, especially when discussion seems to be going round in circles. Giving direct feedback on unconscious behaviour and challenging illogicalities or inconsistencies can move someone on from a position in which they could not previously conceive a way forward. Using this type of confrontation to good effect takes practice; it should be carried out assertively in a calm and supportive manner.

Career counsellors should be well-informed, skilled and offer impartial help. The career counsellor should have a wide base of knowledge of what external resources exist to which clients may be referred for more detailed help or advice about particular jobs or training opportunities.

## How might a career counselling service for doctors be set up?

In one study where 36 key doctors were interviewed to elicit their views about setting up a career counselling service for doctors across a region, there was no consensus between respondents as to who was the best person to provide such services to doctors at different stages of their careers.[4,5] General practitioners and non-medical career guidance experts were both seen as appropriate careers advisers for schoolchildren. Vocational training scheme course organisers were seen as being the most suitable for junior doctors who had decided on a career in general practice, and general practice registrars. General practitioner educationalists skilled in career counselling were viewed as an important resource for those wanting career counselling at all stages of a medical career and were seen as being appropriate advisers for medical students, young and established doctors, pre-and-post-retirement GPs, non-principals and those vocationally trained doctors who have left general practice.

> **The careers service run by the English National Board for nurses is very popular[6]**
>
> The careers network has 2912 nurse members. In a 12-month period to March 1999, the careers service handled 55 902 enquiries and despatched 84 149 items of careers literature. 17 321 enquirers visited the ENB stands at careers exhibitions.

The majority of those interviewed described a vision of a coordinated systematic medical careers service across the region, led by an Associate Adviser responsible for training others and promoting an expert, accessible and available career counselling service in every district. Most wished that all those holding medical educational appointments became more aware of the importance and benefits of career counselling for doctors at all stages of a medical career. Most wanted all those in medical education to have basic career counselling skills and know when and how to refer enquirers on to an expert resource, which might be sited at the centre of the region or as satellites subregionally.

There were just three of the 36 doctors studied who did not share such a vision of region-wide access to career counselling.[4,5] One believed that 'doctors should take responsibility themselves for their own careers and we shouldn't spoon-feed them.' He wanted information about various medical career options to be available on the Internet for anyone to consult if they sought a career variation. Another respondent did not appear to understand the concept of career counselling for qualified doctors at all. The third interviewee was 'not sure if there are careers guidance skills or how good careers guidance experts are'.

The BMA believes that additional funding will be required for providing career counselling services, rather than existing educational funds being re-allocated. The BMA's guidelines envisage careers advisers who are experienced in selection procedures, training requirements, career options and assessing individual doctor's suitability for particular medical careers.[7,8]

The National Association of Clinical Tutors has recommended that the right to receive career counselling should be inserted in junior doctors' job descriptions and educational contracts.[9] The General Medical Council (GMC) has recently specified that pre-registration house officers should have access to careers advice[10].

Postgraduate deans are thought to be well-placed to offer career counselling to trainees or students because of their significant knowledge and experience of a wide range of specialties. It is difficult to imagine deans having sufficient time to counsel more than a handful of doctors. In one region, those requiring career counselling are expected to make their request in writing, accompanied by a curriculum vitae and a brief outline of the problem, so that the request can be directed to the member of the deanery team best placed to help.[11]

---

**Ideas and suggestions for establishing career counselling for doctors in the region were:[4]**

▶ career counselling services should be well-publicised and visible

*continued*

- career counselling services should be properly financed and not run on goodwill as services additional to peoples' current workloads
- a central register of individual people, departments and organisations with specialist interests, skills or enthusiasms to be available resources
- a network of well-informed careers advisers with advertised details about their experience/qualifications, to give those enquiring informed choice about the qualities of potential advisers
- integrate career counselling services into doctors' workforce planning for each district
- include non-medical career guidance experts
- all trainers should be more aware of career development needs of junior doctors and what opportunities there are for future flexible career options
- every established doctor should have the opportunity to reflect with a well-informed adviser on their career progress from time to time to find ways to enhance job satisfaction and prevent burnout
- the careers adviser's personality is more important than their post – they should be motivated and enjoy helping other doctors, approachable, skilled, knowledgeable and capable
- those providing first-line careers advice should know their limitations and where to refer on people and cases outside their own competence
- we need a specialised career counselling resource for poorly performing and sick doctors.

One doctor emphasised the need for specialised career counselling to be available and accessible to poorly performing doctors. This could include a system whereby experienced counsellors eliminate sickness as a cause of the poor performance, consider the under-performer's personality, and provide a series of one-to-one career and progress reviews that take account of any sensitive legal position including registration with the General Medical Council, the handling of any disciplinary procedures and recommendations about fitness to practise.

# Some typical case studies who might present for career counselling

The cases described below are stories drawn from many peoples' experience of advising or counselling doctors. They all require time and help from an experienced career counsellor who is sensitive to their difficulties and career dilemmas. The learning notes capture discussion of these case studies at a series of medical career counselling skills training workshops. The learning points should help would-be careers advisers and counsellors think out what their approaches might be to these complex cases.

Work in trios: you might consider using these case studies yourself in a training workshop in small groups of three, with one person playing the career counsellor, another the doctor being counselled and the third observing the role play. Debrief: take turns to feed back your impressions, how it felt, what you liked or gained, what you disliked or when you felt uncomfortable, angry or upset, and if or when you felt secure about the counselling relationship. Discuss and compare the trios' experiences as a plenary group.

## Gerald: a poorly performing doctor

Gerald is aged 43 years and has been a GP for ten years. After two complaints from patients in the last two years he has been referred by the health authority to the GMC for alleged 'poor performance'. It looks as if they are serious complaints – a failure to visit a terminally ill patient and a late diagnosis of a child presenting with florid signs of diabetes mellitus. The health authority has instructed Gerald to see you, the local GP tutor, to see if you can help. If Gerald doesn't meet you and follow an educational improvement plan while the GMC's performance procedure is underway, the health authority say they will refuse to contract with him for GP services. They tell you confidentially that he is one of the most profligate prescribers in the district and you have wondered about his standards of prescribing yourself when on duty for the GP co-operative and covering his patients.

When you talk to Gerald about his career he says he doesn't really care too much if he does have to leave medicine. But he has no idea what he would do to earn the sort of income his family is used to. He had originally wanted to be a surgeon, but after four years as a surgical registrar and three unsuccessful attempts at the FRCS he had abandoned his hopes. He had then opted for GP training as his wife was tired of moving house and wanted to start a family. Gerald joined his current practice ten years ago. He is the middle partner of a three-man partnership with a list of 8000 patients in an inner-city practice. He works long hours and has had little time recently for continuing medical education or leisure activities.

He is irritated about being asked to see you, arrives late for the appointment and appears rather distracted. How can you as the career counsellor establish a rapport with Gerald and explore his needs?

## Learning notes

Allow sufficient time for meeting to establish rapport and listen to and explore all the issues: at least 60–90 minutes is likely to be required for the first session, with three or more follow-up sessions.

Start sensitively and try to establish a friendly rapport with Gerald, agreeing the purpose of the meeting as a career counselling session. Make it clear that you feel there is no compulsion on Gerald to meet with you, that you are not investigating the complaint and you wish to help him to think through his situation to make a plan for how to proceed.

The counsellor should establish the boundaries and parameters of discussion early on – especially as to confidentiality, if Gerald's continuing to work might threaten patient safety. That is, if as a doctor you know that another doctor is unfit to practise and may be a threat to patient safety you have a duty to inform the authorities about the situation (e.g. the health authority, GMC) if the doctor will not desist from active practice.

Stick with open questioning to establish a counselling relationship, encouraging Gerald to talk by reflecting back his input. Explore the circumstances, constraints, pressures, relationships at work and home in a non-judgemental way.

Use a standard career counselling framework to get Gerald to focus on:

► Who am I and where am I now?
► How satisfied am I with my career and my life?
► What changes would I like to make?
► How do I make them happen?
► What do I do if I don't get what I want?

Gerald should volunteer possible options and think through the consequences of them over the four or so career counselling sessions. You won't get all this done in the first session, when Gerald may take time to let down his guard and be honest with you as the counsellor.

As a career counsellor of a poorly performing doctor you may feel:

► overwhelmed by the problems of the client (stress, alcohol, educational lack, lack of support) and the potential time commitment, and the negativity of the client
► that it is difficult to establish a good relationship with the doctor 'client' because of their initial hostility and suspicion of your role
► that you need much more time than you've got to establish a good relationship
► that it is difficult to be non-judgemental and transmit unconditional positive regard in reality, if you personally have a negative view of their performance or dislike them
► that it takes great skill to stop the doctor client being dependent on you as a counsellor instead of taking responsibility themselves.

## Retaining a high-achieving doctor

Cathy is a 39-year-old GP who works full time in a five-partner practice in a leafy suburb. She has been getting more and more frustrated at work because her partners just won't listen to her ideas for practice developments or delegate responsibility to her for making changes that would benefit them all. She is on the local primary care group (PCG) board but has difficulty getting the others to consider her views even after she has prepared briefing documents and drawn up detailed plans for them.

One of Cathy's hobbies is cooking, and she is considering leaving her GP practice to set up as a cook, teaching cake decorating and hostess cookery while creating her own catering business from home. She has almost finished a Masters in Business Administration (MBA) at the local university and could put her new-found expertise to work with her planned catering business.

### Learning notes

As for Gerald, start by establishing the boundaries of the career counselling session, how long it will last, agree limits to confidentiality, etc. Be aware of using relaxed and positive body language as a counsellor. But be careful not to become 'too friendly' – a medical career counsellor may well feel that he or she identifies with the high-achieving doctor who is consulting them; but if as a career counsellor you breach your counselling relationship by being too friendly you may be less likely to 'challenge' the doctor 'client', and 'challenging' his or her views is one of the strengths of career counselling.

Career counsellors need to realise that their own preferences are not necessarily the same as how others prefer to live their lives at work and home. They should try to get 'under the other person's skin' to understand why others are having difficulties. It is important to know yourself well as a career counsellor to be able to recognise your own underlying prejudices and blind spots which might influence your counselling of others.

Use the same format as for Gerald, moving from 'Who am I and where am I now?' to 'What do I do if I don't get what I want?' as before. Try to establish what will be a successful endpoint from Cathy's perspective and work towards helping her to achieve that. You and Cathy may only take one session to work through her career dilemmas to help her reflect on her situation and plan her future path. Cathy may then develop more insight and understanding to be able to continue to make her own career plans, which might involve staying in her GP practice but adopting a different approach to her partners, moving to a new GP partnership or changing her career in some other way – but not necessarily moving into the catering business.

## How to handle people who feel they are failures

Jane is 41 years old. She had entered medical school as a mature student in her mid-twenties, having left school and worked for eight years. Jane did fairly standard house jobs, a variety of senior house officer (SHO) posts, finally focusing on oncology and radiotherapy. She has been a specialist registrar in clinical oncology for nearly four years and has not yet secured a consultant post despite making three applications in the last year. She is either not short-listed or if she is, a home candidate gets the job. She feels an utter failure, thinks she will never get a consultant job and is wondering about opting for an 'easier' life in general practice or as a psychiatrist. She has come to see you for careers advice to find out how she could swop to another career as she is 'no good' at clinical oncology and thinks she has little chance of getting a consultant's post.

### Learning notes

Set up a good career counselling relationship as before, with similar arrangements and format as for Gerald and Cathy. In Jane's case, you will need to continually remember that career counselling is not about giving direct advice or guidance, which someone like Jane may keep asking for: 'What would you do if you were me?'

Being directive is wrong because direct guidance might:

► absolve people from taking responsibility
► be wrong for that person
► be superficial – decisions made through reflection and experience are more likely to stick and be satisfying
► result in the counsellor being blamed for an inappropriate career path
► be counsellor-centred rather than client-centred.

If a doctor 'client' feels so negative that they cannot describe any 'strengths' about themselves, ask them to recall a time when they did perform well or describe an example when they handled conflict well. Jane will need help realising ways to build up her self-confidence and personal skills. She might choose to learn more about personal management skills rather than attend for a second career counselling session. She might seek out others who have succeeded in gaining the type of post she wants, to hear their tips. Jane might discuss her next application with a senior consultant whose advice she respects, to review her CV, how she promotes herself, the preliminary work and visit she should make prior to a formal interview.

Someone like Jane can always do something even if it is only to change their attitude to their situation. If problems seem overwhelming, the counsellor should encourage the doctor 'client' to choose one issue at a time on which to concentrate.

## How to counsel the transient doctor population at an early stage in their career choice

Robert has just finished his second SHO post in medicine. He is consulting you as you walk into the postgraduate centre together because he knows you have given advice to some of his friends. He wonders what you think of him travelling round the world for a year – will he be able to get back into a hospital job, will travelling spoil his chances of a career, what would you do if you were him? He goes on to explain he cannot decide what he wants to do for a medical career. When he came to university at 18 years old he wanted to be a GP because he had admired his own family doctor so much. But during medical school he wanted to be in whatever kind of specialty he was studying, and must have changed his mind ten times. He wonders if it might be a good idea to work abroad for a while to give himself a chance to know his own mind and get over the break up of his long-term relationship with his girlfriend.

**Learning notes**

If you have too little time or the 'counselling' is done as an informal discussion in a corridor, you will tend to ignore the cues given by Robert about his uncertainty, the break-up with his girlfriend, etc., and you may fall into the trap of being directive. You could gain breathing space by setting Robert some homework to think out the options and then arrange a proper meeting where you both set time aside.

You will need protected time to get him to work through 'Who am I and where am I now?' to 'What do I do if I don't get what I want?', as in all the previous cases. Robert may need your permission to seek further help and be taken seriously.

Your main role with Robert is to get him to reflect on what he wants to do and to think through the pros and cons of different options. You should challenge any limits he puts on his potential or future career plans, and help him decide from where he might seek practical help or gain an inside knowledge of a variety of careers and opportunities.

## How to handle a counsellor's conflicts of interest

Aly has been a GP trainer for ten years and has never had such a difficult registrar as Donald before. There will be a vacancy in the practice soon and the rest of his colleagues really like Donald because he makes them laugh and will want to appoint him if possible. Aly thinks he is not to be trusted but there is no tangible proof. He probably goes home early but is never caught out and always has a plausible excuse for why he was not present that wrong-foots Aly. Donald does make mistakes in patient care but says he'd had inadequate teaching or there were too few resources, etc. – it is never his fault. Donald is now booked in for a tutorial and career planning is the topic for the session.

How should you as Aly conduct the tutorial on reviewing and planning Donald's career when you don't fully trust or like him and feel his performance at work is only just acceptable? Will you give him a reference when he asks you today, especially if it is to apply for a job to work with you? Remember that your other GP partners like him and would be very surprised by your views and suspicions; and any unpleasantness may rebound later if Donald is appointed to the practice.

## Learning notes

This case demonstrates how difficult it is mixing professional development and career counselling in the same session, with the same trainer having three simultaneous roles as educational supervisor, career counsellor and line manager. One solution would be to team up with another tutor or trainer so that they undertake careers guidance or counselling for your trainees and vice versa. It is difficult for trainees to confide in their trainers and honestly discuss their weaknesses or negative feelings about a specialty with someone on whom they are dependent for a reference and maybe patronage.

To make the best of the situation you are in as a trainer with such conflicts of interest, you should be explicit about dealing with each section of the discussion. You should try to distinguish between appraisal, performance development and careers guidance in the same session, and make it clear to your trainee or GP registrar which 'hat you are wearing'. Any difficulties should be resolved in the initial contract setting at the beginning of the session.

If you are going to discuss a trainee's faults, give constructive criticism in a kindly but straightforward way. Keep the criticism factual rather than cast accusations that might lead into dispute around the circumstances or your interpretation. If the counsellor does not have the courage to say what the problem is, the doctor 'client' does not have the opportunity to change.

# References

1 Chambers R (1999) *Survival Skills for GPs*. Radcliffe Medical Press, Oxford.

2 Rogers C (1999) *Client Centred Therapy*. Constable, London.

3 Egan G (1990) *The Skilled Helper* (6e). Brooks Cole, New York.

4 Chambers R (1997) *Need for Careers Counselling for General Practice in the West Midlands Region*. Staffordshire University, Stoke-on-Trent.

5 Chambers R (1998) Careers counselling for general practice. *West Midlands J Primary Care*. **4**: 32–9.

6 English National Board (1999) *Review of the Year 1998–99. Annual Report*. English National Board, London.

7 British Medical Association (1996) *Guidelines for the Provision of Careers Services for Doctors*. British Medical Association, London.

8 British Medical Association (1998) *Medical Careers: a general guide*. British Medical Association, London.

9 National Association of Clinical Tutors (1996) *Training Pack: career counselling, acronyms and abbreviations*. National Association of Clinical Tutors, London.

10 General Medical Council (1998) *The New Doctor*. General Medical Council, London.

11 Paice E and Goldberg I (1998) What do postgraduate deans do? *BMJ Classified, Career Focus*. **6 June**: 2–3.

# CHAPTER 3

# Where are you now – career review and assessment

All doctors should take stock and review their options throughout their careers. Various triggers might occur in your life that prompt you to ask yourself whether you are happy at work, whether you are in the right job and whether it is worth rethinking your present career. Such as when:

(i) faced with a variety of opportunities and options, uncertain of which career path to take

(ii) feeling there is a mismatch between you and your particular medical career – maybe your personal ethics or values are threatened, or your needs and preferences have changed

(iii) feeling demotivated or dissatisfied with your work – maybe your role has changed, or you feel your career has plateaued for too long

(iv) a serious life event occurs – bereavement, marriage, divorce, illness, developing disability

(v) a significant event occurs at work – a complaint from a patient, the death of a patient, a mistake, a critical incident arising from work

(vi) preparing for retirement – wanting to slow down but not stop.

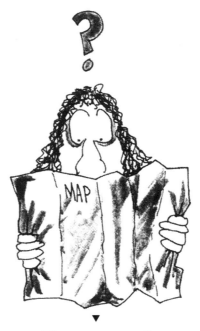

**Where are you now?**

---

**Typical mid-career challenges to reflect on:**

▶ Do you believe you could achieve more?
▶ Are you sure about your future career direction?
▶ Do you want to take control of your career?
▶ Could you make more of the changes in your life – in your personal circumstances, in the NHS?

---

The lack of a clear career structure is a well-recognised source of stress in any workforce and not just medicine. Hospital consultants and GP principals usually work for at least 30 years before retirement once they have gained their senior positions. They may choose to extend their skills, or take on managerial responsibility, but to all intents and purposes they have 'plateaued' in their careers in their mid-thirties.[1]

# Analysing yourself: your skills and strengths, plans and vision

You might do this analysis by yourself or with a mentor, tutor or trusted colleague. You might use the exercises to help someone else.

# Who are you and where are you now?

## Looking inwards

*(i) You*

- What are your strengths and weaknesses as a doctor?
- Do you understand your own personality: have you undertaken a personality profile test?
- What transferable skills do you have that might fit you for a different kind of career?
- How does your current work and life measure up to your inner values?

*(ii) Your current job*

- Do the features of your job fit with your personal style?
- How satisfied are you with your job – working hours, responsibility, location, patient contact, workload, income, challenge, opportunities for change or development, extent of socialising, your skills, on-call commitment, support from colleagues, variety?
- How satisfied are you with your career in general?

## Looking outwards

- What opportunities are there for promotion or other roles in your current job?
- What opportunities might there be for developing new skills or enhancing current skills in your present job?

- What other jobs are on offer elsewhere for which you might apply?
- Have you got enough support from others?

## *Looking sideways*

- How do your current workload and conditions impact on your family?
- How satisfied are you with your lifestyle and the time spent outside work – sport, relaxation, hobbies, travel?
- How much quality time do you have for friends?
- Have you got the work–home balance right?

> Understanding yourself, your strengths and weaknesses, and what you have achieved in life gives you a good foundation on which to build your future.

# Check your skills and strengths

Tick the appropriate column to indicate whether you rate yourself as being competent in these areas at work; add any other items you think are important. Now prioritise which skills need further attention by selecting 'essential', 'desirable' or 'not appropriate' for you or your job.

**Competent**        **Needs attention**
essential/desirable/not appropriate

1 Personal effectiveness

- decision making
- negotiating
- influencing
- motivating others
- winning commitment.

**Competent**          **Needs attention**

essential/desirable/not appropriate

### 2 Personal management skills

- time management
- stress management
- assertiveness
- communication
- networking
- delegation
- presentation.

### 3 Clinical skills

- basic as a doctor
- specialised for your job
- new requirements, e.g. for new role.

### 4 Practical skills

- information technology
- searching for evidence
- health economics.

### 5 Organisational skills

- clinical governance
- patient involvement
- public consultation
- commissioning: what –
- health needs assessment
- establishing new systems: what –
- implementing policies: what –.

### 6 Special functions of your post

- teaching
- research
- managerial.

### 7 Career attainment

- qualifications
- training
- experience.

# What changes do you want to make?

*Where do you want to be in ONE year's time? Write down your goals:*

*Looking inwards*

▸

▸

▸

*Looking outwards*

▸

▸

▸

*Looking sideways*

▸

▸

▸

> ▸ Think widely: academic career, research interest or audit, opportunities for teaching, location, preferences or hobbies, access to relatives, alternative and parallel medical work, availability of cover by colleagues, supportive colleagues, sponsors and friends. Do you know of someone whose career you would like to emulate?
> ▸ Build on your strengths and skills; acquire new skills to develop your full potential. Other roles and experience will add to your skills base. Skills developed outside work may be just as important as those developed as part of your job.
> ▸ How will you know if you have been successful in achieving your goals?

*Where do you want to be in THREE years' time?*
*Write down your goals:*

*Looking inwards*

▶

▶

▶

*Looking outwards*

▶

▶

▶

*Looking sideways*

▶

▶

▶

---

**Thinking of a mid-career change?**

▶ Assess your marketability.
▶ List your transferable skills.
▶ Design a good CV.
▶ Identify unadvertised vacancies.
▶ Contact friends and colleagues through your different networks to explore opportunities and let people know that you are looking for a change.
▶ Scour adverts in different publications: clinical, managerial, higher education, local, etc.
▶ Think widely – seek careers advice, information, guidance and/or counselling.

## How are you going to get there?

Work out the series of steps you will need to take over the next 12 months to achieve your one-year goals; and longer-term action for your three-year goals. Think how to make things happen. To whom can you talk to get more information or advice? Who can you visit to see if their type of work appeals to you? Who can give you well-informed guidance or career counselling?

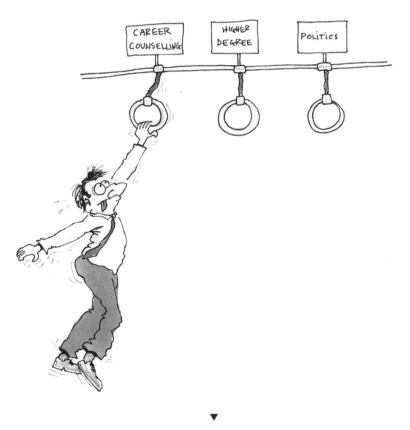

▼

**Career change**

## Getting ready to make a change

*What do you need to do first?*

► Further reflection and review of how satisfied you are with your career, your job, your life in general – as in Stages 1 and 2 and 3.

► Discuss your satisfaction and options with others close to you – at home, your family and friends, work colleagues, trusted advisers and confidantes.

► Find out more information and facts about other careers or new skills.

► Ask someone for advice about opportunities in their field and what their jobs entail.

► Seek careers guidance or career counselling from an impartial careers adviser.

► Make a list of your options and reflect on their relative advantages.

*Are you ready to change?*

► How positive are you about going ahead and making changes?

► Does what you are proposing fit with your ethics, values and boundaries?

► What is it that has limited you from making changes in the past? Have you overcome those constraints or barriers now?

► Are you clear about what interests and motivates you to work effectively?

*So what will you do?*


## Make your plans happen with timetabled action

Think of:

► setting goals
► using your skills and experience
► the timetable

► how you will proceed
► support and resources needed
► overcoming limiting factors.

*So what will you do?*

> Those working for the NHS tend to be tied into staying in the health service by the 'nature of their skills, their socialisation into a particular culture and their pension arrangements'.[1]

# What will you do if you don't get what you want?

Write down your contingency plans.
For instance:

► How could you change your current job so that you have more job satisfaction?
► Re-evaluate your options. What is your 'second choice' alternative career?
► Re-assess your previous goals and objectives?
► What other skills might you develop within medicine or in your leisure time?
► Could you get more balance into your life by building in more self-development time?
► Think if anyone else might help you through all your networks and contacts?
► Can you fit two different jobs into your life, working part-time on each?
► Think again about what you really want out of life.
► Counter self-defeating beliefs.
► Institute better personal stress management.
► Build up your support – at work, with friends, with family and your partner at home.

*So what could you do?*

# Who might help you with your career planning and review?

*Mentor*[2]

A mentor helps the person being mentored (termed 'mentee' here) to realise their potential by acting as a trusted senior counsellor and experienced guide on personal, professional, career and educational matters. The mentor agrees learning objectives with the mentee and subsequently guides them to address their needs, identify their strengths and weaknesses, explore options, encourage reflection and provide motivation. There should be mutual trust and respect in a supportive yet challenging relationship.

A common framework used for mentoring follows three stages:

(i) *exploration*: when the mentor listens and prompts the mentee with questions

(ii) *new understanding*: when the mentor listens and challenges the mentee, recognises strengths and weaknesses, shares experiences, establishes development needs and gives supportive feedback

(iii) *action planning*: encourages new ways of thinking and solutions, agrees goals and decides action plans.

*Buddy*[2]

A buddy is someone in a similar situation to you with whom you have a reciprocal relationship, who gives you unconditional peer support. If your relationship with your buddy is successful you may keep in touch all your working lives. You should each take turns at actively listening to the other, challenging when appropriate, giving constructive and supportive feedback when necessary. Each buddy should trust the other to preserve confidentiality about the issues discussed.

## Supervisor[2]

An educational supervisor works with the learner to develop and facilitate an educational plan that addresses their educational needs. Ideally, educational supervision should be focused on educational development and be separate from supervision of clinical practice or remedial help for under-performance. The supervisor will usually maintain an overview of the learner's performance and career progress.

## Career counsellor[2]

A career counsellor should be non-judgemental and transmit an unconditional positive regard to the person being counselled. A good career counsellor knows him or herself well so as to be able to recognise his or her own prejudices which might influence their counselling of others. A career counsellor should have sufficient insight to be able to understand why other people are having difficulties with their jobs or circumstances. Most doctors do not have the skills to be effective career counsellors without further training.

## Coach[2]

Coaching involves a combination of psychology, business and communication skills. It consists of a partnership between coach and 'client' to clarify the client's goals for work and life and plan how to achieve those goals. Developing self-awareness and insight should lead to lasting change. A coach will focus on building up positive attitudes and behaviour in the individuals being coached.

*Postgraduate Dean or Dean/Director of Postgraduate GP Education, or their deputies: Associate Deans, Associate Directors; clinical or GP tutors, or college tutors*

Deans and Directors of Postgraduate GP Education (DPGPEs) and their senior medical educationalist staff are ultimately responsible for the regional provision of medical careers advice, guidance and counselling for those considering particular careers or contemplating changing their specialties. They are increasingly being asked to help those with career problems, such as failure to progress in a chosen specialty or under-performance. DPGPEs, for example, oversee the management of the 3–5% of GP registrars who either fail or are labelled as under-performing in their training posts.[3]

# References

1   Kent G (1999) Onwards not upwards. *Health Management.* **August**: 20–1.

2   Chambers R (1999) *Survival Skills for GPs.* Radcliffe Medical Press, Oxford.

3   Bahrami J (1999) What do directors of postgraduate education in general practice do? *BMJ Classified, Careers Focus.* **21 August**: 2–3.

# CHAPTER 4

# Structured training for medicine

## General practice

General practice offers a challenging career and despite numerous changes to the structure of the NHS, remains at its centre. There are many career opportunities of a full- and part-time nature. In the past, a trainee's goal was to become a GP principal but recently more doctors are taking up a variety of roles collectively called GP non-principals (for want of a better collective term). General practice is adapting to the changing demography of the workforce, the most recent change being the revamped retainer scheme. 'Portfolio careers', where the working week is made up of more than one type of job, are becoming increasingly popular.

### Training for general practice

The length and content of vocational training is governed by parliamentary regulations. The training programme usually consists of two years in hospital SHO posts followed by one year as a GP registrar in a GP training practice. Regulations do allow for programmes to include up to 24 months as a GP registrar and a minimum of 12 months in hospital posts. Except in the armed forces, where 18 months in general practice is normal, it has not been possible for deaneries to receive funding for anything over one year in general practice due to funding for this component coming from the general medical services (GMS) budget. Following an agreement by the Department of Health and the General Practice Committee of the BMA, the funding will be dispensed from the Medical and Dental Education Levy in the year 2000, just like the SHO posts. This should lead to an increase in flexibility of vocational training schemes with the development of more innovative posts based in general practice.

There is a choice between joining a vocational training scheme (VTS) or of constructing a do-it-yourself (DIY) programme. The proportion of doctors on VTS schemes is increasing because there are advantages over DIY programmes. The benefits are the ability to plan for three years without having to worry about where, or what, the next job will be and guaranteed release to the half-day release course organised by highly trained course organisers, who also act as mentors providing professional support and advice. Study leave is also easier to secure for courses aimed at your future career intention on a VTS scheme, for example attending a family planning course during a paediatric post. Flexibility is often missing on a DIY scheme. These advantages need to be weighed against the flexibility of a DIY programme, enabling SHO posts to be selected to fit in with educational and domestic needs.

Training that follows the standard format is called 'prescribed experience'. At the satisfactory end of training, the Joint Committee on Postgraduate Training for General Practice (JCPTGP) awards a certificate of prescribed experience. The content of prescribed training is dictated by the NHS (Vocational Training for General Medical Practice) Regulations 1997 in England and Wales and the parallel 1998 Regulations for Scotland and Northern Ireland. Doctors whose training does not conform to the requirements laid down in the regulations but consider it to be equivalent, can apply to the JCPTGP for a certificate of equivalent experience. Both certificates are equally valid for a doctor to enter general practice.

## Directors / Deans of Postgraduate General Practice Education (termed 'Dean' in the four London deaneries)

Vocational training for general practice is organised by the DPGPEs throughout the UK. They are usually joint appointments between a university and the civil service. They are experienced GPs who work at a deanery level with a team of enthusiastic course organisers and trainers. Their role is to manage GP training and the continuing professional development of qualified GPs in their area. They select appropriate training posts in both the hospital and general practice phases of training and monitor the standards of training provided for trainees.

## The Joint Committee on Postgraduate Training for General Practice (JCPTGP)[1,2]

The JCPTGP was set up in 1974. It is an independent body composed of members of the General Practice Committee of the BMA and the Royal College of General Practitioners (RCGP), with representation from other bodies including the UK Conference of Postgraduate Advisers in General Practice, the Association of Course Organisers and GP registrars. It is the competent authority in the UK for GP training under 'Title VI of EEC Council Directive 93/16/EEC'. Its main responsibilities are to set the standards of GP training throughout the UK and the armed forces, monitor the provision of training courses in the deaneries and the approval of posts used for GP training. It issues certificates of prescribed and equivalent experience to doctors who have satisfactorily completed the required training for general practice and exemption certificates for those with acquired rights.

## Prescribed experience

In order to obtain a certificate of prescribed experience, applicants must supply documentation to the JCPTGP which confirms that they have satisfactorily completed at least 36 months' full-time or part-time equivalent training within seven years of application for a certificate in posts approved by the JCPTGP. At least 12 months must be as a GP registrar. For applicants whose employment began after 30 January 1998, all components of summative assessment must be passed.

The programme of training must include neither less than six months nor more than 12 months in each of two of the following specialties:

- general medicine
- geriatric medicine
- medical paediatrics
- psychiatry
- one of A&E, general surgery, A&E and general surgery or A&E and orthopaedics
- one of obstetrics and gynaecology, obstetrics or gynaecology.

Experience in other relevant specialties may also contribute to a maximum of six months towards the overall training period.

Summative assessment comprises an assessment of factual knowledge (an MCQ examination), an assessment of written work (an audit project), an assessment of consulting skills (usually by analysis of a video tape of the doctor's own consultations), and a structured trainer's report of the doctor's knowledge skills and attitudes.

## Equivalent experience

Applications for a certificate of equivalent experience are considered by the JCPTGP on an individual basis. The doctor is expected to demonstrate a well-balanced training experience equivalent to that needed for a prescribed certificate. Applicants must also complete 12 months' training as a GP registrar within a total period of training of not less than 36 months full-time equivalent. Summative assessment is also compulsory if training began after 30 January 1998.

## Acquired rights

This is a specific term used under the European Directive that enables member states the right to grant certain doctors the right to practise as GPs without the need for a certificate of vocational training. In the UK, they are all doctors who:

▸ were already a GP principal in the NHS or in the armed forces on or after 15 February 1981 and before 31 December 1994

▸ worked as an assistant (or on the retainer scheme) or deputy (including locum) in NHS general practice on either 10 separate days in the four years or 40 separate days in the ten years ending 31 December 1994; they hold an acquired right to work in either of those capacities but are not a principal

▸ hold a recognised primary medical qualification awarded in an EEA state other than the UK and were established in the UK on 31 December 1994 as a fully registered medical practitioner because of that qualification, which is recognised in the UK by virtue of the Medical Directive or other enforceable community right.

The acquired rights term under Title IV of the European Directive 1993/16/EEC of 5 April 1993 has caused considerable problems recently with the case of Spanish-graduated doctors. There have been many Spanish doctors who had to have their training stopped because of this directive. Any Spanish doctor who was awarded their primary medical qualifications in Spain before January 1995 has acquired rights to practise as a GP anywhere in the UK. As a consequence they *cannot* take up a GP registrar training post, despite their lack of GP training comparable with a UK graduate. The lack of clarity in the regulations has disappointed many young doctors. It is important that anyone contemplating training in general practice should clarify their status with the JCPTGP and a DPGPE.

## The future of GP training

Training to be a GP has always been a compromise between education, training and providing a service to patients. While the training of specialists has appeared to be a national priority with the development of Calman's higher specialist training, many believe that the system for training future GPs is in need of urgent attention. There are, however, the first signs of a new dawn. Funding streams for GP training are to be unified in England. There are similar changes happening in Scotland, Wales and Northern Ireland. The General Practice Committee, DPGPEs and the RCGP are working together to improve the management of training, which should lead to more flexible and exciting training programmes based on principles of adult learning. The system whereby training practices could advertise for registrars is being replaced by an enhanced management system that should improve recruitment and selection based on the principles of equal opportunities. Flexible training opportunities should also increase. Hopefully this is the start of a revolution in general practice education which will enable the development of programmes of learning being based more on the needs of doctors wishing to pursue a career in general practice, rather than hospital medicine. It is also hoped that there will be a period of higher professional education available to all after the completion of their training programmes. The future is very exciting!

In the past, advertisements for vocational training schemes and for GP registrar posts in training practices have been placed in medical journals by local trainers and course organisers. In future, the DPGPEs will manage recruitment arrangements. This will lead to different arrangements for recruiting to the general practice training programmes; details are still to be announced. Up-to-date information is available from DPGPEs and information about local schemes will continue to be available from the VTS course organisers. A comprehensive guide to training is being published by the Department of Health.

## *The nature of general practice*

### The role of the GP

The NHS was founded in 1948 and has undergone many reorganisations since then, culminating in the most recent developments of PCGs and primary care trusts (PCTs). It has, however, continued to keep GPs at its heart. The vast majority of first contact healthcare occurs in general practice in the UK, resulting in an average four or five contacts per patient per year with the GP. Nearly 90% of all decision making takes place in primary care with only 13% being referred on to secondary care. General practitioners have increasingly worked as part of wider primary health care teams (PHCTs). The composition of a team varies slightly depending on local circumstances but usually includes nurses, health visitors, practice managers, secretaries and receptionists. Many teams include community midwives, physiotherapists and social workers. PHCTs work together to provide direct and accessible personal and family care to the local population over many years. Their role is not just to cure disease and relieve symptoms but to promote health and prevent disease and disability. General practitioners also have a key role as gatekeeper to secondary care hospital services.

### The GP principal as an independent contractor to the NHS

General practitioner principals form the largest group of senior doctors in the NHS. They are independent contractors, that is, self-employed people who have a contract with their local health authority. They exercise freedom in how to run their own practices. It is this freedom that has allowed flexibility and adaptability which has led to innovation and the rapid development of general practice with consequent improvement in patient care in many areas of the UK.

With freedom comes responsibility. Standards of service provided do vary, with many NHS managers arguing that the means of control of an employer are lacking. The demise of fundholding and the advent of PCGs and PCTs should address these concerns. But even if GPs' independent contractor status remains, increased budgetary control may reduce flexibility and stifle innovation in the new circumstances.

Dentists, opticians and pharmacists also have an independent contractor status with the state. This independence is highly valued by GPs as it allows them to act as patients' advocates. It does, however, result in complications in the way they are paid. The NHS pays the GP a gross income. This includes a component towards the practice's expenses including staff salaries and the cost of premises in addition to providing for a net income. The target income is set by the government after receiving a report from the Doctors' and Dentists' Review Body, who in turn have taken evidence from any interested parties, but importantly from the profession, the Health Departments and from surveys conducted at the request of the Review Body. It is a complex system that protects the independent contractor status but can lead to anomalies and inequalities.

GPs receive set allowances each year, one for each patient registered with the practice, one for undergoing some continuing medical education and one that increases with seniority or length of service. They then claim fees from the health authority for each item of core work that they do, such as child immunisations and cervical smears. Certain other non-core work such as minor surgery also attracts a fee. An inefficient system that fails to submit claims for work done will affect the profits. Since the profits must pay overheads and the staff salaries, any shortfall affects GPs' take-home pay. All regulations regarding terms and conditions of service and the contract those in primary care have with the health authority are laid out in the Statement of Fees and Allowances (know as the 'Red Book').[3,4]

## Hours of work – availability to patients

General practitioners should normally be available at times and places approved by their health authority. Patients must be informed of the availability. Full-time GPs should be available for not less than 26 hours of patient contact time per week. Availability is normally for five days in a week for at least 42 weeks per year. This can be reduced to four days per week if the doctor is involved in health-related activities. The hours should be convenient to patients but the health authority cannot stipulate which days the GP should be available.

It is obvious that GPs work far in excess of these hours of contact with patients but the 1990 contract attempted to assure patients of uniform access to GPs across the UK. Out-of-hours cover is the responsibility of the GP but is increasingly delegated to others as part of GP co-operatives or deputising services.

## *Flexible working in general practice*

Flexible working is a broad term covering a variety of working time arrangements and patterns. It can include school term-time working, part-time work, shift work, job-sharing or casual work. Hours may fluctuate with service demands.[5] One of the main stimuli to increasing the flexibility of working arrangements has been the increased proportion of women entering general practice. Women GP registrars now outnumber men. Women make up 27% of the full-time equivalent workforce, a rise of 4% since 1991. An increasing number of men are also following the trend of flexible working.[6]

> **Trends in UK GPs' work commitment[6]**
>
> ► trend to part-time GP working (95% full-time in 1990, 85% full-time in 1997)
> ► falling full-time female GP trend (84% full-time 1990, 63% full-time 1997)
> ► rising number female GP job sharers (3% in 1990, 5% in 1997)
> ► rising number half-time female GPs (2% in 1990, 14% in 1997)
> ► rising number three-quarter-time female GPs (11% in 1990, 18% in 1997)
> ► rising number part-time [half or three-quarter-time] male GPs (2% in 1990, 5% in 1997).

## Part-time GP principals

Doctors wishing to work part time as a principal can work in a partnership with a contract for either fewer than 26 but not fewer than 19 hours, or fewer than 19 but not fewer than 13 hours.

Doctors wishing to become part-time GP principals are encouraged both nationally and locally by health authorities but it depends on the practice's own organisation as to how the duties and hours are divided, which can lead to inequity and frustration. Flexible working patterns require flexibility from GP partners as well as the doctor concerned. The success of innovative working arrangements depends as much on the willingness and attitudes of everyone involved as on the structure itself.

## Job sharing[7]

It is also possible to job share for 26 hours a week. The popularity of job sharing is slowly increasing, 5% of male and female GPs have made such an arrangement.[6] This normally involves two people sharing one full-time post; usually but not necessarily with a 50:50 split of hours, tasks and pay. The two 'job-sharer' GPs must receive at least one-third of the income of the highest-earning partner between them, although this may be divided unequally between the two sharers. Some job-share partners divide the week in half, others do half of each day. Sometimes job sharers deputise for each other over holiday or sickness absence periods. Such job-sharing posts often come as a way of a full-time principal reducing their hours for personal or professional reasons, but sometimes a pair of doctors submit a joint application for an advertised post. Many regional offices of the BMA or health authorities will help doctors seeking potential job-share partners and hold personal details on a database.

---

**The part-time GP principal**

DB works all day Tuesday, Wednesday afternoons and on call at night, Thursday until mid-afternoon and an occasional Saturday morning. She finds she has more commitment to the practice than when she was working as a locum in various practices. She enjoys the continuity of care as a contrast to her previous locum work. In her practice, she and the other two GPs work very independently from each other with their own following of patients.

---

## Retainer scheme

The doctors' retainer scheme was introduced in 1969 to allow doctors taking a career break to stay in practice on a part-time flexible basis. It has been available in both hospital and general practice. There are about 700 doctors on the retainer scheme in the UK; most are women doctors and almost all are in general practice. The general practice retainer scheme was updated in June 1998.[8] The change in regulations permitted practices to employ a doctor on the retainer scheme for up to four sessions per week. The local health authority reimburses the practice £45.75 (as at 1999–2000 prices) towards the retainer doctor's salary for every 3.5 hour, half-day session. A fee is paid to the retainer doctor to cover some of the costs of membership of a defence society and subscription to a professional journal. A doctor can remain as a retainer for a maximum of five years but the region's DPGPE can extend this in exceptional circumstances. Practices employing retainees must be either an approved training practice or specifically approved by the DPGPE. They must be capable of providing adequate education, supervision and support. The scheme is popular and the numbers have risen dramatically since the scheme has been revised.

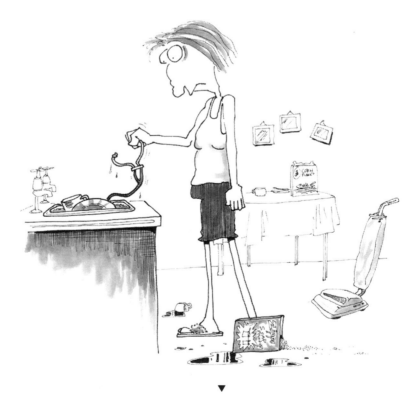

▼
**The retainer scheme**

**The retainee**

GH does four morning surgeries followed by up to two home visits per week. The surgery times fit in well with taking the children to school. Previously she worked as a locum and then as an assistant in her current practice until the new retainer scheme arrangements rendered it financially advantageous to her practice for GH to transfer on to the retainer scheme. She likes being a retainer, feeling it enables her to keep up to date without taking on as much of a commitment to the practice as being a GP principal would entail.

## Salaried GPs

Salaried posts are becoming more common because of the development of Primary Care Act Pilots. In these pilot sites, salaried doctors are employed with a specific remit, such as providing extra care for the homeless, relieving inner-city GPs or practising in areas where it is more difficult to recruit GP principals. Associate schemes also exist to provide relief for single-handed GPs in remote areas.

**The salaried GP**

RW is employed by a trust as a salaried GP working in a deprived inner-city area on a renewable yearly contract. He has a relatively small list size which generates a higher-than-average consultation rate. His terms of service cover pay, hours and conditions, which exclude out-of-hours working; his list of patients receive out-of-hours care from the other GPs in the practice to which he is attached, who are reimbursed by the trust for providing emergency cover.

**Locums**

These are doctors who are employed by other GPs to assist on a temporary basis. There are many long-term locums who work with some practices and deputising services for many years. They must have a JCPTGP certificate or have acquired rights to practise as a GP. Doctors taking up a new post as a locum, assistant or deputy must satisfy their employer that they are eligible to work in that capacity. A certificate of acquired rights is not necessary but the JCPTGP will issue one if a doctor requests that eligibility is demonstrated.

---

**The locum**

TM has been working as a GP locum for the last year. When he finished his vocational training scheme he wanted to take his time finding the right practice in an area in which he wanted to live and work. He has made several applications but as yet has not found the right partnership. He likes to be in control of his working hours and no longer wants to work over nights or weekends, preferring to spend the time with his family. He feels that his experience of working as a locum in so many different practices means that he has a better idea of what he wants from his future GP partnership and the kind of service he wants to offer as a GP principal.

---

**The National Association of GP Non-Principals**

This association was formed in 1997. Its aim is to represent all GP non-principals to ensure equality with principals and reduce the isolation of the practitioners. The association has been very active, politically and educationally. They act as a resource for all matters relating to non-principals and have organised educational meetings, promoted the development of local groups and produced a handbook that includes an excellent personal professional development planning section.

# Higher specialist training

Since the publication of the report of the working group on Specialist Medical Training in 1993,[9,10] training in hospital medicine has been extensively revised.

## The Specialist Training Authority (STA)

The STA of the medical Royal Colleges is a joint organisation with representation from the GMC, Postgraduate Deans and the Royal Colleges, and patient representatives. It oversees all training posts and is responsible for maintaining standards of training and awarding the Certificate of Completion of Specialist Training (CCST) – the passport for membership of the specialist register and entry to the consultant grade. Individual colleges produce syllabuses and assessments and inspect training posts but the STA is responsible for ensuring all college activities comply with the requirements of the legislation.

A CCST can be awarded in two specialties if an approved training programme has been followed in both, for example, in radiology and nuclear medicine. Subspecialty training is usually undertaken before award of a CCST and after completion of the full training programme, and can be added to the entry in the specialist register.

In order to work towards a CCST the doctor needs to apply to the Postgraduate Dean for a national training number (NTN). This is usually awarded after successful competitive entry on to a specialist rotation and will then stay with the trainee until the programme has been completed. These numbers were introduced to aid educational, financial and workforce planning and management. The reforms to the specialist training system have, however, had teething difficulties and in some fields numbers of specialist registrars do not yet match the consultant jobs available.

Equivalent numbered posts exist for overseas trainees as visiting training numbers (VTN) and fixed-term training numbers (FTN). The latter are also available for trainees with a CCST who are undergoing subspecialty training.

## Specialist registrars

This new combined training grade has replaced the registrar and senior registrar grades. Specialist registrars will have undergone a period of general professional training and basic specialist training as a senior house officer of around three years, and will spend a total of seven or eight years working towards their CCST.

## Terms and conditions

Since April 1996, doctors in training grades have been employed by their trusts. But the national terms and conditions of service for hospital medical and dental staff still apply. A full-time working week is 40 hours paid at the basic rate. Additional periods of duty are contracted for one of three types of schedule – full shifts (when the maximum hours per week must not exceed 56 hours), partial shifts (which are 64 hours per week) or with an on-call rota (72 hours per week). All of these additional duty hours are paid at less than the basic rate.

NHS trusts have the power to determine their own consultant contracts and terms of service. Full-time consultants work 11 notional half-days of three and a half hours and may not earn more than 10% of their gross NHS salary from private practice. Maximum part-time consultants are paid ten-elevenths of the full-time salary and have no such restrictions on private practice.

## Other specialist hospital appointments

### Staff doctors

The staff grade was introduced in 1988 under the *Achieving a balance*[11] proposals which aimed to improve the career structure and meet the service requirements by offering a permanent non-consultant career grade. It can be entered into from the SHO grade but is often staffed by experienced doctors who do not wish to take on the responsibility of a consultant post. They are popular in 'overcrowded' specialties, such as obstetrics and gynaecology, and orthopaedics. Staff-grade doctors may take part in the specialist registrar on-call rota but they do not have continuous responsibility for patients.

These doctors are responsible to a named consultant and fulfil a service requirement. Promotion prospects are limited to associate specialist after four years; but staff-grade doctors in some deaneries are being given the opportunity to enter the final year of a specialist registrar training grade to allow them to qualify for a CCST.

### Associate specialists

These are personal appointments created when there is a pressing service need which does not require a new consultant post, or where doctors already working in the hospital meet the criteria for a permanent position but have not been able to reach consultant status for personal reasons. They are senior posts and the post-holder shares the consultants' rota rather than the junior doctors' rota. Status and delegation of duties are negotiated locally.

It is possible for these doctors to get back on to the training ladder if they wish, with some credit being given for experience as well as for qualifications.

### Clinical assistants

These posts were initially created to enable GPs to work for a small number of sessions in hospital with the aim of developing or maintaining a special interest. GPs with sufficient expertise may be upgraded to a hospital practitioner, a more senior grade for those with postgraduate qualifications in the field. Clinical assistantships are now held by any doctors who may work up to five half-days – although some trusts offer contracts for more sessions. They are often held by women with families who want a career break.

### Trust doctors

These posts were created to fulfil service need in hospital trusts at different levels in the hospitals; their job descriptions and terms and conditions vary considerably. They may undertake service work that is equivalent to that of a SHO or SpR, but they are not training posts.

## Flexible training

Three years after qualifying, two-thirds of women doctors and a quarter of men want to train flexibly. By this stage, one in five of the doctors qualifying three years before had spent time outside the NHS, often working abroad or travelling.[12]

According to the Department of Health rules, flexible training is open to any male or female doctor who has 'well-founded' personal reasons for wishing to train flexibly, such as responsibility for dependants, ill health or disability. Eligibility must be confirmed with the postgraduate dean before applying for a flexible training post.

The UK does offer a limited number of flexible training placements for a variety of specialties. About 10% of specialist registrar posts are part-time, varying from 18% in psychiatry to 3% in surgery. Part-time training in hospital medicine is at least a half-time commitment under European Law. The UK is one of only two European countries with an under-supply of doctors (–0.9% medical unemployment) and this, the long training periods in the UK and the relatively high population to doctor ratios in the UK have fuelled the need to establish flexible training schemes to retain as many doctors as possible.

Training for general practice can be completed flexibly. Doctors wishing to train flexibly are actively supported by the DPGPEs. It is advisable to consult the DPGPE when considering flexible training because there are differences between hospital and GP training that need to be considered, especially by doctors constructing their own scheme. European regulations state that GP training must not be less than 60% of full-time and must contain at least one week of full-time work in both the hospital and general practice components. Although easy to organise, the regulations have caught out some doctors in the past who have not declared their desire to train for general practice and have completed a half-time post only to have difficulty getting the experience approved.

A survey of flexible trainees in the UK in 1998,[13] found that 777 of the 797 respondents were women doctors. Almost 75% were higher specialist trainees (specialist registrars, senior registrars or registrars); the rest being SHOs. Most were in their early- to mid-thirties, with about 10% being aged under 30 years and 12% older than 40 years. The most common reason to have applied for flexible training was responsibility for children, cited by 89% of respondents. Most (738) lived with a partner; 26 were single parents. The pattern of contracted basic hours per week was: 28 hours (15%), 24 hours (52%) and 20 hours (17%); in addition, the average contracted on-call commitment was 15 hours per week. Two-thirds of respondents reported regularly working more than their contracted hours, the average additional time worked being four hours per week.

There are no formal schemes for part-time house officer and SHO posts. Individual arrangements need to be discussed with the flexible training advisor (every deanery has one for each specialty) and application made to the chosen hospital in open competition. The specialist registrar grade does have formal flexible schemes. Entry is by competitive interview and trainees will need a NTN or VTN. Specialist registrars already working full time can transfer to flexible training programmes and vice versa.

The budget for flexible training is held by the deanery and hitherto the number of flexible general practice trainees has been hindered by financial complications. Some deaneries are now keen that this money can move with the trainees into general practice registrar posts.

# Guidance for overseas doctors

The UK actively welcomes doctors who wish to train in the UK. There is a long tradition and the benefits to both the overseas doctor and this country are well-recognised. There are, however, rules that need to be observed. This section seeks to guide you through a potential minefield of regulations. It does not seek to be a comprehensive list, but will introduce you to them so you should seek further information.[14]

## European Economic Area countries

A recognised primary qualification from a European Economic Area (EEA) member state will give automatic registration with the GMC. For European nationals after full registration, specialist training requirements are exactly the same as for UK graduates and a CCST at the completion of training will be recognised in all member states.

A fully registered doctor with a specialist qualification from a member state gains automatic entry to the specialist register. Even within the EEA, however, mutual recognition of specialist qualifications varies from one college to another and can be bureaucratic; contact the appropriate colleges for advice. An EEA national has no need for an immigration visa.

## Definition of an overseas doctor

An overseas doctor is a person who, regardless of where their primary qualification was obtained, does not have a right of indefinite residence or is not settled in the UK (as determined by immigration and nationality law) or who does not benefit from European Community rights or who is not a national of the EEA.

## GMC Registration

Overseas doctors who want to train in the UK must hold and maintain registration granted by the GMC. This may be Provisional, Limited or Full Registration if the doctor wishes to train in the hospital or community health services. Doctors wishing to train as a GP registrar must hold Full Registration. The requirements for Registration vary depending on the country of graduation. The exact criteria are published by the GMC.

## The Professional and Linguistic Assessment Board (PLAB) Test

Many overseas doctors are required to pass the PLAB Test before becoming eligible to apply for GMC registration. It includes an Objective Structured Clinical Examination. In 1997, there were 3612 attempts at the PLAB test of which 1318 (36%) passed. It is held 14 times a year in the UK; Part 1 can be taken abroad. The structure of the exam is currently under review. The examiners are looking for standards of written and spoken English and clinical knowledge that would be expected of a SHO, but it is interesting that the medical press recently reported that in a validation exercise in 1998, only two of the 50 UK doctors taking the examination passed it.[15]

Doctors taking the test are not eligible for employment, they can enter the UK as visitors and are required to produce evidence from the GMC or a test admission card before they are granted leave to enter the UK. It is normally granted for a period of six months.

## Leave to enter the UK

A doctor who does not satisfy immigration or nationality law requires leave to enter the country. In order to secure leave to enter, conditions may be imposed; these may include limiting the period of stay, restrictions or prohibition of employment, etc. These are endorsed in the doctor's passport or travel documents. One of the requirements for leave to enter is that the doctor is eligible for appropriate GMC registration.

## Immigration rules

The Immigration Acts of 1971, 1988 and 1996 regulate entry into and the stay of a person in the UK. Major changes for doctors and dentists wishing to train in the UK came into effect from 1 April 1997. The essence is the period of permit-free training.

## Permit-free training

This is a special provision under the immigration rules where overseas doctors can enter the UK for the purpose of post-graduate training in hospital or community health services without a work permit. Not all training grades are eligible for work permits. Provisions for general medical practice are different.

To qualify, a doctor must satisfy the immigration authorities that he or she has the appropriate GMC registration, intends to leave the UK on completion of his or her training and is able to maintain and accommodate him or herself and any dependants without recourse to public funds.

The type of training being undertaken determines the duration granted.

- Pre-registration House Officer employment – there is an initial grant of 12 months and provision for an extension to cover illness, etc.
- Basic Specialist or General Professional Training – this covers SHO posts. The initial grant is no longer than three years with provision for an extension to a maximum of four years.
- Fixed Term Training appointment (FTTA) (Type II programme) – this is for doctors seeking a limited period of postgraduate basic or higher specialist training. The duration of the fixed training period is usually granted, but this fixed training period is often shorter than three years.
- Higher Specialist Training (Type I programme) – the period granted is initially for three years. This can be extended for up to another three years depending on the requirements of their training programme.
- GP Training – the rules are different to hospital training and are explained in more detail below.

The Home Office takes into account advice from the Post-graduate Dean before making extensions to the initial period of permit free training.

**Opportunities for training within the specialist registrar grade**

There are two types of training programme to which overseas doctors may be appointed. These are:

Type I – a higher specialist training programme that leads upon satisfactory completion to a CCST.

Type II – a higher specialist training programme or Fixed Term Training appointment (FTTA) which is an agreed training programme that usually lasts for six months to two years that does not lead to a CCST. These programmes are restricted to overseas doctors without a right of indefinite residence or settled status in the UK or EEA nationals but not to UK nationals unless they already hold a CCST.

All doctors are also candidates for locum appointments for training (LATS) which offer similar opportunities for training and locum appointments for service (LAS) which are not training opportunities.

The NHS operates an equal opportunities policy. The Postgraduate Dean is responsible for operating the appointment process (except for LAS). All appointments are through open competition.

## The Overseas Doctors Training Scheme (ODTS) – 'sponsored' postgraduate doctors

The overseas doctors training scheme (ODTS) was established in 1984 for those doctors who are not nationals of the EEA or who do not hold a primary qualification obtained in the EEA. The scheme is organised by the Specialist Royal Colleges with support from the medical education department of the NHS Executive.

The numbers of doctors entering the scheme in 1997 under the sponsorship of the various Royal Colleges ranged between 15 via the Royal College of Ophthalmologists to 123 via the Royal College of Physicians. Most doctors on the scheme have already obtained postgraduate qualifications in their home countries.

The GMC will grant *Limited Registration* without need to take the PLAB Test, provided it is satisfied that the applicant has the necessary knowledge skill and experience and that the doctor will pursue supervised postgraduate training in an approved post or programme. Exempt doctors must pass the required test of English language, the International English Language Testing System (IELTS) language test run by the British Council.

It is possible for a sponsored doctor to work in the SHO grade or in a Type II programme in the SpR grade (FTTA). Transfer from the SHO grade to the SpR grade depends on evidence of satisfactory progress and a review by the Postgraduate Dean with advice from the UK sponsoring doctor and the Royal College.

## Appointments in academic or research medicine

Doctors wishing to study, train or work in universities or other academic or research institutions may enter the UK under the following categories:

▶ *Visitor*: period not exceeding six months. Employment is prohibited. Eminent doctors will normally be allowed to enter as visitors for up to 12 months without the need for a work permit.
▶ *Work permit employment*: employed appointments.
▶ *Permit-free employment*: for posts that combine academic or research activity with postgraduate clinical training. An honorary NHS appointment in a hospital or community health service training grade is needed to enable the doctor to be employed by the university.

## Training for a career in general practice as an overseas doctor

The eligibility and funding for training in general practice in the UK are different to hospital practice.

## Immigration status

Overseas doctors who are seeking to train or practise in the UK or EEA need to establish their immigration and employment status as, except under exceptional circumstances, there is no funding available from the NHS for training in the GP registrar year. These immigration rules do not apply to EEA or a family member who is entitled to enter or remain in the UK by virtue of the provisions of the immigration (EEA) order 1994. There is no sponsorship scheme for general practice training.

The rules are rather confusing, because if an overseas doctor wants to train in general practice in the UK they need to be in possession of a Training and Work Experience Scheme (TWES) certificate. But under a standing agreement with the Department of Health and the Overseas Labour Service, a TWES certificate would not be issued to doctors wishing to train as GP registrars.

There has been considerable confusion over these rules. It is important to remember that overseas doctors who are training in hospital posts may not automatically be able to obtain a post as a GP registrar on completion of their hospital posts. They should, therefore, check their eligibility well in advance of the date they wish to take up a post.

## GMC registration for GP training

All doctors working or training in general practice in the UK must have full GMC registration. This has caught out doctors who are working in hospital posts and assume that they can transfer into a GP registrar post on limited GMC registration. It has also caused considerable difficulty for overseas and EEA doctors wishing to do Pre-registration House Officer posts (PRHO) – they cannot because only full registration is acceptable and this can only be awarded after successful completion of their intern or PRHO year.

*Further information may be obtained about overseas doctors' training from*:

- Postgraduate Deans: each Deanery has one. There is usually an Associate Dean working with the Postgraduate Dean, who has particular responsibility for overseas doctors. Details of addresses of Postgraduate Deans are obtainable from the NHS Executive Medical Education Unit.
- 'Guide to Immigration and Employment of Overseas Medical and Dental students in the United Kingdom', published by the Department of Health (1998). For copies telephone 0800 555 777.
- NHS Executive, Medical Education Unit, Quarry House, Quarry Hill, Leeds LS2 7UE.
- The Home Office, Immigration & Nationality Department, Lunar House, Wellesley Road, Croydon CR5 4BY.
- Overseas Labour Service, W5, Moorfoot, Sheffield S1 4PO.
- The Medical Information Officer, National Advice Centre, The British Council, Medlock Street, Manchester M15 4AA.
- The General Medical Council, 178 Great Portland Street, London W1N 6JE.

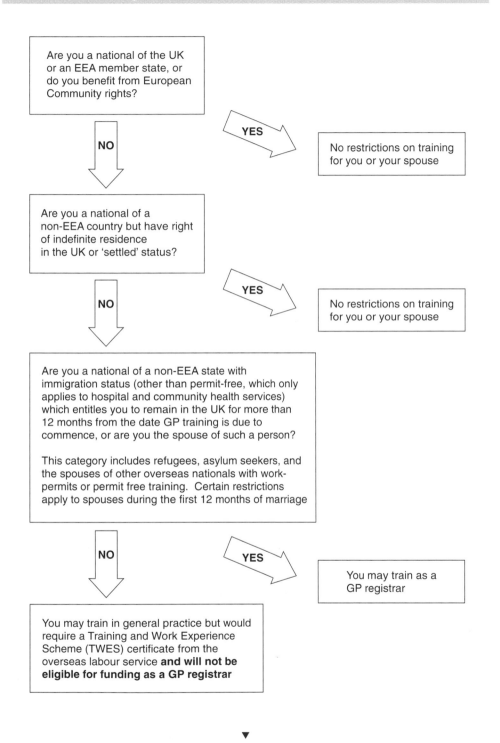

Figure 4.1: Flow chart: eligibility to train as a GP registrar in the UK

# References

1  Joint Committee on Postgraduate Training for General Practice (1998) *A Guide to Certification*. Joint Committee on Postgraduate Training for General Practice, London.

2  Joint Committee on Postgraduate Training for General Practice (1998) *Recommendations on the Selection and Re-selection of Hospital Posts for General Practice*. Joint Committee on Postgraduate Training for General Practice, London.

3  Department of Health (2000) *Statement of Fees and Allowances (The Red Book)*. Department of Health, London.

4  Ellis N and Chisholm J (1997) *Making Sense of the Red Book* (3e). Radcliffe Medical Press, Oxford.

5  Bigrigg A and Monaghan A (1999) Flexible working in family planning and reproductive health care. *Br J Fam Plann*. **25**: 33–4.

6  Department of Health (1998) *Statistics for General Medical Practitioners 1987–1997*. Bulletin 1998/16. DoH, London.

7  Norfolk Health Authority (1993) *Job Sharing in General Practice*. Health Authority, Norfolk.

8  NHS Executive (1998) *HSC 1998/101*. DoH, London.

9  Calman K (1993) *Hospital Doctors Training for the Future. Working party on specialist medical training*. DoH, London.

10  Department of Health (1998) *A guide to Specialist Registrar Training*. DoH, London.

11  Department of Health (1987) *Hospital Medical Staffing: achieving a balance*. DoH, London.

12  British Medical Association (1999) *Cohort Study of 1995 Medical Graduates*. BMA, London.

13  Norcliffe G and Finlan C (1999) Attitudes to flexible training. *BMJ Classified, Career Focus*. **13 March**: 2–3.

14  Department of Health (1997) *Guide to Immigration and Employment of Overseas Medical and Dental students in the United Kingdom*. DoH, London.

15  News Editorial (1999) *Doctor*. **10 June**: 11.

# CHAPTER 5

# Career paths

Given the paucity of informed careers advice and the small numbers of people taking an interest in giving such guidance, it is hardly surprising that some young doctors end up as 'square pegs in round holes'. Deciding on posts that will suit their personality and aspirations from the myriad opportunities (some books give up to 80 alternatives within medicine) can be daunting. Facing the fact that the wrong choice was made requires even more courage.

This chapter is in three parts, giving information to help answer three types of question:

**Alternative tracks: what are some of the more popular fields of medicine?**

**Branching tracks: what other options allied to medicine might appeal?**

**Parallel tracks: what are the jobs that might contribute to a portfolio career?**

Much of the material presented here was obtained from surveying a cohort of doctors who graduated in 1988. Asking them to describe their career choices helped to define the more popular routes available within medicine. The personal 'case histories' of some of these doctors give a flavour of what it means to work in these fields. Some of the views expressed are composites of conversations with more than one doctor in order to give a balanced view. Some of these conversations lasted for up to an hour. The enthusiasm with which interviewees participated is explained by one comment from a retainer in general practice: 'I really got to where I am now by default and had to make it up as I went along. There didn't really seem to be anywhere you could go to find out about career choices. I was told by one consultant it would be a waste if I entered general practice because I was too clever! I'm glad I ignored that as he turned out to be totally wrong. Once you are in the world of general practice there is a whole network of people who can help, but you don't know about that until you get here. Most junior doctors are totally drained after house jobs and can't even think straight. Anything that helps people make better choices must be a good thing.'

Information and addresses are given as a starting point. You will need to contact the organisations given for full details and insider information or some of the other sources of information[1] such as those given in the Appendix.

## Alternative tracks: what are some of the more popular fields of medicine?

### Accident and Emergency medicine

| | |
|---|---|
| General professional training: | Two years as SHO with experience in A&E and at least one other specialty. |
| Entry requirement: | MRCP, FRCS, FRCA. There is a specific version of the FRCS for those interested in A&E. |
| Higher Specialist Training: | Five years. Research is important but a higher degree less so. Teaching and management skills are expected. Fellowship of the Faculty of A&E Medicine. |

Career opportunities:    Becoming more popular now training
                         is structured. There are 420 consult-
                         ant posts and 185 training posts, of
                         which 22% are held by women. There
                         is currently a shortage of people to fill
                         available consultant posts.

Faculty of Accident and Emergency Medicine, Royal College
of Surgeons of England, 35–43 Lincoln's Inn Fields, London
WC2A 3PN. *Tel*: 020 7405 7071.

JM is a consultant in A&E.

'I always wanted to be a surgeon since I was a boy, and I went
straight from house jobs on to a surgical rotation. I realised
that I liked the challenge of the unknown in A&E so after I
got my Part 1 FRCS I opted for that. The mix of the life-
threatening and the trivial is nice, and you meet all sorts of
people. The only drawback is that there can be a lack of
continuity sometimes. We patch them up and send them on
and someone else watches their progress.

   Part of my job is to organise teaching for the casualty officers
and the GP trainees, and I did a part-time, distance-learning
certificate in teaching. When I was in training I think people
made it up as they went along – but now teaching and education are better organised and the trainees get a better deal.'

SB is a GP with a clinical assistant post in paediatric A&E.

He constructed his own vocational training scheme, which
included a year of paediatrics, during which time he took the
Diploma of Child Health (DCH). When he left the Children's
Hospital he was offered the opportunity to come back as a
clinical assistant in A&E. He initially left hospital medicine
and did locums as a GP.

'When I found a partnership one of the other GPs was also a
clinical assistant in another casualty department, so I took up

the offer to work there. I work one afternoon a week, the salary is paid into the practice and we organise the cover for the practice between us. It's an ideal opportunity for a GP. The hospital likes employing GPs because they think pragmatically, order fewer investigations than casualty officers and have more experience of family medicine. From my point of view I see more trauma and orthopaedics than I would in practice. It is certainly more interesting than five days a week in general practice.'

## Anaesthetics

| | |
|---|---|
| General professional training: | Minimum of two years as a SHO including 21 months in anaesthesia and three months in intensive care medicine plus at least six months in a post other than anaesthetics. |
| Entry requirement: | Primary FRCAnaes. |
| Higher Specialist Training: | Five years. FRCAnaes completed after first year. A special interest or skill such as pain relief is more important than research. Might need to spend some time working in intensive care because specialist posts for training are less common. |
| Career opportunities: | Flexible training and flexible working are major features, as is the large number of posts – 2960 consultants and 1441 training grades. Passing Part 1 FRCAnaes with a year in approved posts qualifies the doctor for the Diploma (DA), which can lead to sessional work in private practice such |

as for ECT in psychiatric hospitals. Sessional work and non-consultant work such as clinical assistant posts make it attractive as a part-time career.

Royal College of Anaesthetists, 48–49 Russell Square, London WC1B 4JY. *Tel*: 020 7813 1900.
Association of Anaesthetists of Great Britain and Ireland, 9 Bedford Square, London WC1B 3RA. *Tel*: 020 7631 1650.

AI has been an associate specialist in anaesthetics for two years.

'I started out training in anaesthetics and got my first part [of the previous college exam] after three years. A staff-grade post came up in my hospital after just a year of higher specialist training, during which I got my FRCA. This meant I could settle in the area where my husband was also working and stop travelling around. I was in effect coming in to do my sessions and going home. The on-call duty was only once a fortnight and it suited us really well. After four years as a staff grade I was 'promoted' to Associate Specialist. I run the pain clinic and have limited managerial responsibility, which makes it a bit more interesting without overloading me with administration. I work four days a week and it is a 9–5 day with no on call, which is very civilised!'

---

**Pros and cons of anaesthesia as a career[2]**

*Plus points*:

- ► sociable occupation: you will interact and work with all disciplines
- ► you can put personal leadership skills to good effect
- ► good for people with an interest in gadgets
- ► good if you enjoy the buzz from emergency work and functioning under pressure at times.

*continued*

*Minus points*

▸ the job can be unpredictable and wreck your plans for out-of-work activities
▸ the pressure and demands of the job are stressful
▸ an anaesthetist can feel isolated at times taking responsibility for major decisions without peer support.

## Care of the elderly

| | |
|---|---|
| General professional training: | Two years as a SHO in various medical specialties. |
| Entry requirement: | MRCP. |
| Higher Specialist Training: | Six years. No exit exam. |
| Career opportunities: | A growing field, only 700 consultant posts at the moment but increasing at more than 40 per year, reflecting the concerns over an ageing population. A diploma of geriatric medicine offers some training for general physicians or GPs with an interest in the speciality. |

British Geriatric Society, Royal College of Physicians, 11 St Andrew's Place, Regent's Park, London NW1 4LE. *Tel*: 020 7935 1174.

CA has been a consultant in care of the elderly for two years.

'I did a six-month casualty post at first while I was applying for jobs, then I got a three-year general medicine rotation. I followed that with nine months as a SHO in neurology and medicine for the elderly during which I passed the MRCP.

I then got a national training number and a three-year specialist rotation in medicine for the elderly.

People often talk about how the population is ageing but what that actually means is that half the population now survive beyond 75, mostly in reasonable health. In fact much of my work is just like general medicine. The obvious differences are degenerative conditions like dementia or stroke if issues of long-term care arise, because then the job involves a co-ordinating role as advocate for the patient. We have a large rehabilitation service and much of what I do is to sort out social issues.

Recently there has been a lot of interest in end-of-life decisions and sometimes it is necessary to reassure relatives that you will continue to treat patients properly while at the same time trying not to let intellectual curiosity get the better of you and lead you to intensive investigations and intervention.'

## Clinical pharmacology

| | |
|---|---|
| General professional training: | At least two years of general medical training. |
| Entry requirement: | MRCP. Post-membership subspecialty experience, e.g. oncology, infectious disease or cardiology, is an advantage. |
| Higher Specialist Training: | Lecturer post with honorary registrar status in department of clinical pharmacology. Secondment to industry or protected time for research can be built in depending on individual interest. Exit routes include Diploma in Pharmacological Medicine (Royal College of Physicians) and the CCST, becoming a member of the Faculty of Pharmaceutical Medicine. |

Career opportunities: The main career choices are the pharmaceutical industry, which has its own career structure and posts at all levels for doctors, or academic and regulatory posts such as in medical schools and the Committee on Safety of Medicines. Some general physicians have training in pharmacological medicine as a special interest and can become affiliated members of the Faculty.

Faculty of Pharmaceutical Medicine of the Royal College of Physicians, 1 St Andrew's Place, Regent's Park, London NW1 4LB. *Tel*: 020 7224 0343.

JB is 43 and medical manager of a major pharmaceutical firm. He initially trained in pharmacy and went to work as a product manager in a drug company following completion of an MBA. He then went back to university, qualified as a doctor and, following jobs in general medicine, took the Diploma in Pharmaceutical Medicine. He worked as a clinical research physician for two years and became an associate member of the Faculty of Pharmaceutical Medicine before working his way up inside the industry.

'My original plan was to be a GP but political changes to the health service put me off. Then after house jobs I was totally worn out and thought there had to be something more to life. The pharmaceutical industry is short of good doctors at the moment so it is quite a good time to join – these things go in phases. I think it is also viewed a bit more positively than it has been in the past, as a positive career choice rather than a last resort! I am starting to rethink my career again now and it seems there is a bit more two-way traffic of doctors back into the health service than there has been previously, you used to burn your bridges if you left. If anyone is thinking of the pharmaceutical industry a good grounding would be a couple of years doing phase I trials in a clinical trials unit. It's a good way to get an insider's view of different companies and is a gentle introduction because it's very clinical and you still wear a white coat!'

## Clinical radiology

| | |
|---|---|
| General professional training: | There are no SHO posts in radiology, candidates will have a minimum of two years postgraduate experience but usually more up to registrar level, plus the MRCP. A good understanding of anatomy is essential, MRCS may help. |
| Entry requirement: | None, but very competitive entry. |
| Higher Specialist Training: | Five years. First year is non-clinical with very little service commitment and no on call as candidates study for the FRCR part 1. Research is built into the training scheme. Post-FRCR fellowship strongly encouraged, often with travel abroad. |
| Career opportunities: | The sessional nature of many posts means this specialty lends itself to flexible training and working. There are consultant vacancies in most fields. It is calculated that each physician or surgeon needs the support of one-third of a radiologist. Imaging techniques are advancing and demands on the specialty are growing. |

Royal College of Radiologists, 38 Portland Place, London W1N 3DG. *Tel*: 020 7636 4432/3.

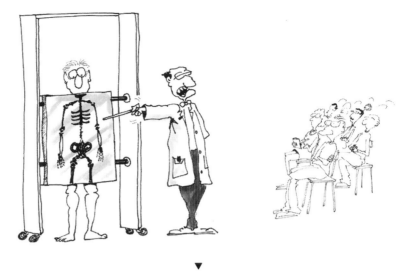

Clinical radiology

> **Why become a radiologist?[3]**
>
> The good bits ...
>
> ▶ well-structured training schemes
> ▶ popular and expanding specialty with a high profile
> ▶ good career prospects
> ▶ diverse job with opportunities to work in many different
>   fields and with a broad range of imaging modalities
> ▶ key role in solving diagnostic dilemmas
> ▶ combines intellectual and practical challenges
>
> ... outweigh the bad bits,
>
> ▶ the FRCR exam
> ▶ retraining in a new specialty
> ▶ no overall control of the care of the patient.

*Dermatology*

| | |
|---|---|
| General professional training: | Minimum of two years as a SHO in general medicine. |
| Entry requirement: | MRCP. |
| Higher Specialist Training: | Four years. Some experience in related fields, such as dermatological surgery, genetics, genito-urinary (GU) medicine, oncology or infectious diseases, is expected. No exit exam. |
| Career opportunities: | Although this is a small field and seen by many as a 'cinderella specialty' it is well-organised and expanding rapidly. It is largely an outpatient specialty with little on call. Twenty percent of consultant posts are held by women. There are two Diplomas in Dermatology; the one from the University of Cardiff is a distance-learning package. Many GPs take this as well as some dermatology registrars looking to improve their career prospects. |

British Association of Dermatologists, 19 Fitzroy Square, London WIP 5HQ. *Tel*: 020 7383 0266.

MS has been a consultant in dermatology for six months.

'This is an extremely competitive field, with a bottleneck at SHO level – there are only 50 specialist registrars in the country. Once you have a training number the posts are matched to consultant numbers so career progression is assured from that point on. The good thing is that there is no exit exam. You need the MRCP to get into training, but then that is all.

I was a SHO and registrar in general medicine for nearly five years before I decided on dermatology, but that was all good experience. The most useful job I had was in oncology. It can be extremely busy in outpatients but the lack of on-call work more than makes up for that.'

## Genetics

| | |
|---|---|
| General professional training: | Minimum of two years as a SHO in general medicine and preferably paediatrics as well; often much more. There are no SHO posts in genetics. BSc or MSc in genetics are common and research registrar post an advantage. Many enter after higher specialist training in another specialty, such as paediatrics. |
| Entry requirement: | MRCP or MRCPCH. |
| Higher Specialist Training: | Four years for those with no genetics experience. |
| Career opportunities: | Excellent opportunities for research especially in molecular techniques. There are only 67 clinical posts in the country, 40% are held by women. |

Clinical Genetics Specialist Advisory Committee, Royal College of Physicians, 11 St Andrew's Place, Regent's Park, London NW1 4LE. *Tel*: 020 7935 1174.

Genetics is very much a clinical specialty with a requirement for good communication skills. Geneticists are involved with diagnosing and predicting congenital disorders and must be able to discuss risk and counsel families. There may be close contact with colleagues in obstetrics and paediatrics as well as general medicine.

CH is a consultant in clinical genetics.

'It took much longer than I would have liked to get here but perseverance seems to be paying off. I started out on a medical rotation as a SHO and after I passed the MRCP I joined a paediatric rotation and was successful in the DCH and the MRCPCH. During that time one of the posts was combined with a clinical geneticist and I started to get really interested in the particular difficulties of counselling families with inherited disorders.

I registered for a MMedSci and transferred to a genetics specialist training scheme. It was a bit of a circuitous route but all the experience has paid off. I think that time spent in a paediatrics job is particularly worthwhile.'

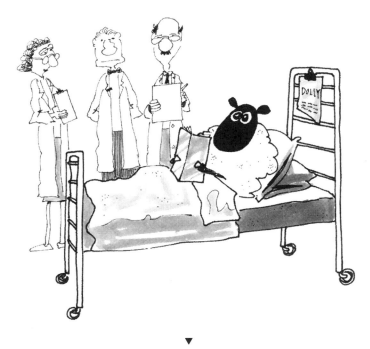

▼

**Genetics**

## Genito-urinary medicine

| | |
|---|---|
| General professional training: | Two years minimum. For those with MRCP six months must be in obstetrics and gynaecology (O&G), or gynaecology. For those with MRCOG a minimum of one year in acute medicine, with on call. |
| Entry requirement: | MRCOG, MRCP. |
| Higher Specialist Training: | Four years. Integral part of training is the in-patient care of patients with HIV, as is training in contraception, counselling skills and epidemiology. |
| Career opportunities: | This is a field with opportunities for flexible career patterns. Possession of a CCST leads to a consultant post but there are many staff grade and associate specialist posts in community GU clinics. Clinical assistant posts are common. Another advantage is sociable working hours, on call is rare. Community clinics are increasingly the site of clinics such as colposcopy, infectious diseases and vulval clinics. |

Medical Society for the Study of Venereal Diseases, Royal Society of Medicine, 1 Wimpole Street, London W1M 8AE. *Tel*: 020 7290 2900.

CM is a consultant in GU medicine having originally wanted to do O&G.

'I trained in obstetrics and gynaecology with a special interest in psycho-sexual medicine. After several years of one-in-two and one-in-three rotas, I got "burnt out" frankly. I wanted to get married, hopefully have children and be able to see them at weekends.

MRCOG is a much better entry qualification to have for this specialty than MRCP, although it is the latter that most people tend to have. So long as you have some experience in infectious diseases, rheumatology and dermatology, gynaecology training is far more useful. There are very good career prospects, once you have got a training number the positions are matched to consultant posts. It's very much like general practice in many ways, the patients by and large self-refer and I never know what the next patient will walk in with. The unknown can be quite exciting. The only difference is that we don't have background notes on the patient. Sometimes they have just got off a plane from Africa. Infectious disease experience is very important; a large part of my work is with HIV-positive patients.'

## Obstetrics and gynaecology

| | |
|---|---|
| General professional training: | One year as a SHO in O&G and a year elective in two fields such as neonatal paediatrics, urology or endocrinology, though psychiatry is also popular. |
| Entry requirement: | Part 1 MRCOG. |
| Higher Specialist Training: | Five years. MRCOG completed after two years usually. One year of research and a completed MD seems to be essential. Some subspecialty training in the sixth year in oncology, uro-gynaecology, infertility or feto-maternal medicine/ high-risk obstetrics helps find jobs that are increasingly specialised. |

| Career opportunities: | Highly competitive with the recent changes to structured training creating a bottleneck just below consultant level. There will be 253 post-CCST trainees by the end of 1999. Good opportunities for private work for those interested, but busy nights and high work load are common. Eighteen percent of 1040 consultant posts are held by women; 39% of training posts are held by women, with 8% working part time. |

Royal College of Obstetricians and Gynaecologists, 27 Sussex Place, Regent's Park, London NW1 4RG. *Tel*: 020 7771 6200.

JJ, 34, is a specialist registrar in O&G.

'I was originally on a vocational training scheme for general practice. Then when I was doing O&G I decided to specialise. I already had the DCH from my paediatrics job so that counted towards my sabbatical period. I would not advise anyone to come into O&G as a career at the moment. The work is interesting but there is a total bottleneck at specialist registrar level. Someone really messed up the numbers when the unified grade was introduced so there are too many doctors with the CCST looking for consultant posts. Maybe in a few years time it will be better.'

## Occupational medicine

| General professional training: | Two years SHO or GP vocational training. |
| Entry requirement: | None, though many candidates attend a postgraduate training course for |

occupational physicians leading to the Diploma of Occupational Medicine (multiple choice paper and submission of portfolio). The Associate of the Faculty of Occupational Medicine requires experience of working in the specialty for 18 hours per week over six months or equivalent, and includes a written, oral and clinical examination as well as a portfolio of work. The MRCGP or MRCP is desirable but not essential.

**Higher Specialist Training:** Four years. Membership of Faculty of Occupational Medicine by exam and research dissertation.

**Career opportunities:** This is one of the fastest-growing specialties in the NHS, where consultants also look after the health needs of employees. But there are also posts in all the armed forces, in universities, in industry and public bodies such as police and fire services. Positions within the Health and Safety Executive as advisory inspectors to industry also exist. Part-time opportunities are extensive and about 3000 doctors hold part-time posts, mostly GPs with no formal qualification, although an increasing number now have the Diploma.

Faculty of Occupational Medicine of the Royal College of Physicians (Training Body), The Society of Occupational Medicine (Continuing Professional Development), 6 St Andrew's Place, Regent's Park, London NW1 4LB. *Tel*: 020 7487 3414.

Institute of Occupational Health, University of Birmingham, Edgbaston, Birmingham B15 2TT. *Tel*: 0121 414 7854; *Fax*: 0121 471 5208.

LM was a principal in general practice for four years and is now an occupational health physician for a car manufacturer.

'When I started in general practice the partnership was responsible for undertaking one session a week at a local factory as the medical officer. I took over the position and decided to study for the Diploma of Occupational Health. Eventually I decided to leave general practice to go into occupational health full time. That was just when the changes in Higher Specialist Training resulted in training schemes and I was allocated a national training number. Most of the faculty-approved posts are attached to industry and quite isolated and my trainer did not even work where I worked. But there is a day-release scheme and the newsletter, *Occupational and Environmental Medicine*, keeps you in touch and advertises jobs.

It is a very interesting job. Parts of the job are not that different from general practice – you deal with some of the same things – but since I am at the factory it prevents the workers needing to have time off. The balance is different and you have to remind yourself that you are on the side of the patient not the employer if you discover a health problem that could potentially put his or her job at risk. The other thing about the job is consistently reminding the company that you are a doctor and not just a health and safety officer. But that is one of your responsibilities, to check that the workers are not at risk from chemicals, etc.'

**Occupational health services include:[4]**

- assessments for fitness to work
- pre-employment medicals
- statutory health surveillance
- health screening
- health promotion
- pension fund evaluations
- rehabilitation advice
- advice on compliance with health and safety law.

**Areas of occupational medicine in which GPs can obtain training:[4]**

- diagnosis of occupational diseases
- occupational hygiene – measurement and control of dust, fumes, noise, etc. in the working environment
- toxicology
- epidemiology and statistics
- ergonomics
- environmental medicine
- health and safety law
- fitness to work
- rehabilitation.

## Orthopaedic surgery

| | |
|---|---|
| General professional training: | Minimum two years as a SHO in general surgical specialties as well as plastic surgery and neurosurgery. Often an anatomy demonstrator post. |
| Entry requirement: | MRCS (previously FRCS). |

| Higher Specialist Training: | Six years. FRCS(Orth) after four years. Study for an MSc or MD is not essential but training in a sub-specialty is. Training is onerous and the on-call commitment especially in trauma or accident surgery can be very demanding. |
| Career opportunities: | There are 1300 consultant posts in the country and only 20 of them are held by women. It is a competitive field but career progression is good. The bottleneck is at the bottom of the specialist registrar grade, often requiring experienced surgical registrars to become SHOs in orthopaedics. NTNs are linked to consultant posts. |

The Royal College of Surgeons of England, 35/43 Lincoln's Inn Fields, London WC2A 3PN. *Tel*: 020 7405 3474.

PA is a senior registrar in orthopaedics and trauma. She took a straightforward route through being an anatomy demonstrator to SHO posts.

'I always wanted to be a surgeon, and as soon as I did my first SHO post in orthopaedics I knew it was for me. I have never found any barriers or discrimination and it is a complete myth that you need to be physically strong. We have power tools now and it is all about technique. It is a very busy job, I have never done less than a one in four on call and I never see my husband, but I feel the rewards are worth it. I suppose one of the main barriers may be the lack of role models. You hardly ever see a female surgeon let alone an 'orthopod'. But you have to just decide if it is for you and go for it.

There is no real requirement for research as yet – it's probably one of the few fields where you don't need an MD to get on.'

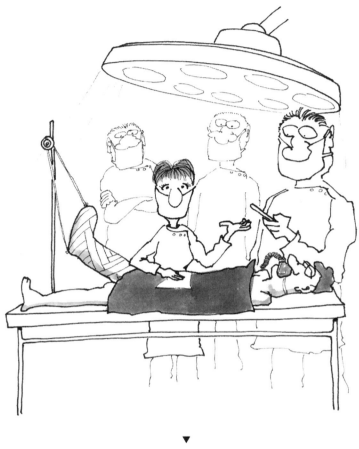

▼
**Orthopaedic surgery**

## Paediatrics

General professional training:

Minimum two years as a SHO with six-month posts in paediatrics and neonates.

Entry requirement:

MRCP or MRCPCH.

Higher Specialist Training:

Five years.
Study for an MSc, usually part time, is encouraged.

Career opportunities:     Every grade in this specialty has an on-call commitment. Community posts are often included in the local hospital on-call rota. There are currently 1300 consultants, 35% of whom are women. Fifty-three percent of the training grades are held by women, with 15% working part time. Flexible training is a reality. Recent rapid expansion in community consultant positions means that there are sometimes fewer candidates than posts.

Royal College of Paediatrics and Child Health, 50 Hallam Street, London W1N 6DE. *Tel*: 020 7307 5600.

CJ is 39 and a specialist registrar in paediatrics. Following a BSc in zoology, he spent time as a hospital porter waiting to get into medical school. He followed his own GP vocational training scheme, gained the DCH and decided that he wanted to specialise in paediatrics. His consultant advised him to finish vocational training, including the registrar year in general practice, but after achieving his JCPTGP certificate, he applied for a paediatric rotation. He passed the MRCP, completed higher specialist training and in six months will have his CCST.

'I have had no objective careers counselling so far, but the advice to finish GP training was good even though it was given in a spirit of incredulity that someone as "old" as me would want to change course! I had a grounding in different specialties and general practice was good experience in family medicine. I believe that general practice can be whatever you want it to be but the pace of hospital medicine suited me better.'

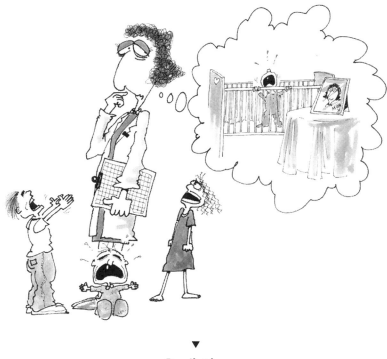

**Paediatrics**

*Palliative medicine*

General professional training: Must include 12 months acute general medicine.

Entry requirement: MRCP, MRCGP, FRCA, FRCR (clinical oncology).

Higher Specialist Training: Four years. No exit exam.

Career opportunities: Rapidly expanding (10% increase in consultant posts per annum). Largely outside the NHS, charitably funded. Fifty percent of consultants are women.

Association of Palliative Medicine of Great Britain and Ireland, 11 Westwood Road, Southampton SO19 1DL. *Tel*: 01703 672888.

AR is 36 years old and has been a consultant in palliative medicine for two years. She originally followed a vocational training scheme and after passing the MRCGP examination became a part-time partner in general practice. After a year or so she started work as a clinical assistant in a local hospice for one session a week. Increasingly interested in palliative care, she decided to leave general practice and was accepted on to a higher specialist training rotation for palliative medicine. Four years later she was granted a CCST and now holds a joint NHS consultant and hospice medical director post.

'I definitely feel that my time in general practice has helped me. There is a lot of teamwork in palliative care and you learn to rely on the nurses and listen to the relatives. That's very similar to general practice, so my time as a GP gave me a good grounding.

It was a bit of a leap though to leave a GP partnership and the job security, but on call is not busy and that made a nice change. As a consultant I am not on call now and the juniors are rarely called. My one piece of advice to others would be to get good experience in general medicine and do some anaesthetics if possible. Palliative medicine can be an emotionally draining specialty but the rewards in terms of job satisfaction are worth it.'

### Pros and cons of palliative medicine[5]

*Plus points*:

- retain much patient contact during training and when a consultant
- integrate with all hospital disciplines and GPs

*continued*

> ▶ work as part of a supportive multidisciplinary team
> ▶ well-structured training
> ▶ opportunities for flexible training and flexible careers
> ▶ opportunities to influence service development
> ▶ good quality of life.
>
> *Minus points*:
>
> ▶ emotionally challenging and demanding
> ▶ constantly dealing with great uncertainty
> ▶ can be professionally isolating
> ▶ few opportunities to develop an academic career.

## Pathology

| | |
|---|---|
| General professional training: | General medical experience at SHO level recommended for at least two years. |
| Entry requirement: | MRCP required for some fields and gives an exemption from one year of higher specialist training. |
| Higher Specialist Training: | Four years leading to MRCPath. MD useful as research is strongly encouraged. Training is subspecialty-specific. Five fields: histopathology, chemical pathology, microbiology, immunology and haematology. |
| Career opportunities: | Excellent prospects especially in histopathology, where consultant expansion has exceeded the number of doctors completing their training. All spend some time in the lab but have a greater or lesser clinical input depending on personal interest. |

Royal College of Pathologists, 2 Carlton House Terrace, London SW1Y 5AF. *Tel*: 020 7930 5861.

AB is a medical microbiologist. Most microbiologists do a general medicine training including infectious diseases, chest medicine, paediatrics or GU medicine before specialising in pathology. The MRCPath exam cannot be taken until 2–3 years into the rotation and an MSc is advisable. Career progression in medical microbiology at the moment can be difficult. Only 13 new consultant jobs are available each year and by the end of 1999 there was already a backlog of at least 34 post-CCST trainees. The Royal College of Pathologists estimates it will take 3–4 years for the backlog to clear under the new training guidelines. It is worrying that 50% of trainees are in rotations that do not have College approval so they will also find jobs hard to come by at the end of training.

'Clinical experience is essential. I did a SHO rotation in medicine and passed the MRCP and it was a very good grounding. I then did a six-month infectious diseases job and studied for the Diploma in Tropical Medicine and Hygiene. You would be surprised how much tropical medicine there is in Southampton! That was when I really decided on the specialty. I like the academic aspect of the job, the rigorous evidence base to the discipline, and the fact that if you read well and keep up to date you can speak authoritatively because the evidence is there. I admit that the less onerous on-call requirement was also a factor. It is much less arduous than general medicine. It is the kind of field where you can actually have a life outside work. Apart from the career progression I would advise any one to give it a go, and even that will sort itself out in time.'

**Attractions and drawbacks of pathology[6]**

'It's not all dead bodies and microscopes.'

Attractions:

- ▶ combines science and clinical practice
- ▶ rapidly advancing subspecialties
- ▶ provision of essential services
- ▶ good career prospects
- ▶ excellent training programmes
- ▶ limited on call
- ▶ application across the whole of medicine
- ▶ multidisciplinary working environment
- ▶ opportunities for pure and collaborative research.

Drawbacks:

- ▶ misunderstood by many – the back room image
- ▶ often under-resourced
- ▶ involvement in and responsibility for laboratory management (although this is an attraction for some).

## Psychiatry

| | |
|---|---|
| General professional training: | Three years SHO. General medicine encouraged. |
| Entry requirement: | MRCPsych. |
| Higher Specialist Training: | At least three years, subspecialty or general rotation. Professional training is well-established and organised; attendance at day-release schemes is common for all the training grades. |
| Career opportunities: | One in eight consultants in the NHS is a psychiatrist and career progression can be rapid as there is a shortage |

of consultants at present. Candidates should expect to be part of a multidisciplinary team and often the structure is less hierarchical than in other specialties. Career options are varied and flexible.

Royal College of Psychiatrists, 17 Belgrave Square, London SW1X 8PG. *Tel*: 020 7235 2351.

MG has been a consultant forensic psychiatrist for 18 months. At medical school he could not decide between anaesthetics and psychiatry and so he did 18 months as a SHO in anaesthetics first to 'try it out'. Some of that time was spent anaesthetising for ECT and eventually he switched to his other career choice. He started a rotation in psychiatry, then became a senior registrar in forensic psychiatry. He has an MSc in Criminology and the MRCPsych.

'I work with a clinical assistant in the prison service who is also a GP so you can see there is a lot of flexibility in psychiatry. As a profession it is very open to people who have done other things. Two years ago, following the government review of the service, the number of secure units was increased, creating a lot of new consultant jobs, and career progression was quite rapid. It's slowing down a bit now but it is still good.'

CD has been a clinical assistant in psychiatry for four years. Following full-time structured training in general adult psychiatry she passed the MRCPsych. She then took the decision to leave the career grade and take a clinical assistant post.

'It was an easy decision for me because it was more suitable for the family. There was no on-call commitment and I worked for six sessions a week. With two children 17 months apart it was ideal; I wasn't really free to do research about other careers. What made it more difficult was that everyone I spoke to said it was a bad idea. They seemed to think I was "selling myself short". All the consultants thought I should be a consultant, as though it was the only career option.

Recently I have started to wonder if I have failed to reach my full potential and I am discussing the possibility of converting the post to that of an associate specialist. It gets harder every time a new senior registrar comes and I have to explain myself again. I don't think that any doors have closed to me because I left after I had passed the membership exam. I could even go back to higher specialist training in the future if I want to as I have the experience.'

## Child and adolescent psychiatry

This subspecialty of psychiatry deals with childhood illness, which can be very rewarding to treat. It is currently an under-subscribed specialty with vacant consultant places. Training follows a distinct path after general professional training, but in addition some general psychiatric rotations have paediatric posts. It is helpful to have done a SHO post in paediatrics and even to have taken the DCH exam, as childhood development plays a key role in understanding child psychiatric conditions. Be prepared to see distressing cases of child abuse.

Some trainees find it useful to have undergone personal psychotherapy, but that is not a compulsory part of the training. Child psychiatrists do, however, need to be able to communicate well with children and parents. They must be able to think logically, deal with uncertainty and cope with complex, multifactorial problems that may be insoluble.

Many child psychiatrists work part time and it is a career that combines well with family life.

**Clinical experience required during specialist registrar training for child and adolescent psychiatry[7]**

Inpatient, day patient and outpatient experience of all child ages, including pre-school children and adolescents. Experience covers emotional disorders, educational difficulties, paediatric liaison work in emergency situations, as outpatient consultations and long-term cases.

- child guidance unit
- conduct disorders
- learning disability
- disorders associated with physical illness
- neuropsychiatric problems
- forensic work
- work with residential establishments outside the NHS.

## Public health medicine

| | |
|---|---|
| General professional training: | Three years in recognised training posts. A few SHO posts in public health medicine exist but they are rare. |
| Entry requirement: | MRCGP or MRCP. |
| Higher Specialist Training: | Five years. Training varies from region to region but includes a Masters in Public Health (MFPHM) by examination after two or three years. |
| Career opportunities: | Only 343 consultant posts in the NHS; 36% are held by women with 17% part time. It is clearly an epidemiology-based specialty and can tend to be a management-only post. Communicable |

disease control is a branch that may bring some patient contact that may otherwise be lacking. Health authorities, regional offices, government departments and academic departments are other sources of employment.

Faculty of Public Health Medicine, 4 St Andrew's Place, Regent's Park, London NW1 4LB. *Tel*: 020 7935 0243.

HJ is a consultant in Public Health Medicine who originally trained as a GP. He wanted some time to do some research and applied for a full-time MSc course in communicable diseases. Following that, and after a period doing GP locums, he decided not to go back into practice but to put his new research and epidemiological skills to use by joining a public health higher specialist training rotation that led to MFPHM.

'When I was at medical school I always found myself rather more interested in diseases than patients. Patterns of health and the way things affect populations was what drew me into this field I suppose. Now that I am here of course it is a great opportunity to actually make a difference. I think people think we sit by the phone waiting to advise on when to give immunisation against varicella in pregnancy, but there is a bit more to it than that! I work in communicable disease but cancer registration is another popular field and of course there is a lot of scope in policy and administration. We work very closely with the health authority, especially around immunisation policies. All sorts of people can be successful in this field but all will need good people skills, communication skills and a certain rigorous approach to best evidence.'

JH is a medical adviser to a health authority and public health physician.

'After eight years in general practice and some contact with the managers running our local GP hospitals, I could see that the growing ability of British general practice was not matched by an understanding of that potential by NHS managers. Public health medicine offered a means of using my experience of patients and the NHS to influence decision making at a higher level.

Of course it is not as simple as that. There is a five-year training programme with a range of challenging and stimulating subjects. It is a difficult specialty to pin down but its richness partly derives from being able to put together widely varying skills to help sort out complex problems.

Public health medicine has a common interest with general practice in that both need a population perspective. Being able to understand the needs of patients and clinicians gives a totally different quality to decisions compared to those of managers. You need to take a longer-term view and be able to accept that influencing the lives of a larger number of people can be as fulfilling as the direct care of individual patients. Influencing the causes of ill health may mean that you do not see direct outcomes of your actions but the opportunity exists to change things on the grand scale.'

## Branching tracks: what other options allied to medicine might appeal?

### Academic medicine and research

In an ideal world, the natural curiosity of those brightest A-level students who enter medical school would lead to questioning and investigation throughout their careers. More often than not, research is seen as a necessary stepping stone in their career progression. Everyone can benefit from developing skills in critical reading, essential for the reflective practitioner.

Some doctors are bitten by the research bug and enter academic medicine where teaching and research play a greater role than individual care. University departments, the Post-graduate Dean and Royal Colleges are the best sources of advice. Training programmes and degrees exist on a part-time and full-time basis. For those leaving the NHS the pharmaceutical industry is an excellent source of training and experience.

Funding for most people will not be in the form of a research training fellowship from a single body but come from a competitive tender to charities and other funding bodies such as the NHS Executive Research and Development Directorates.

Undergraduate teaching goes alongside research in academic units. Most teachers are not trained as teachers but there is increasing pressure from the Royal Colleges and the Post-graduate Deans that this be addressed. There are Masters pro-grammes in medical education at the Universities of Dundee, Cardiff, Nottingham, Wolverhampton and Staffordshire but many universities have generic higher and professional edu-cation qualifications and often now train their lecturers internally. The National Institute of Teaching and Learning offers membership to those who complete a programme in education.

*Alternative training routes to*:

1 Research fellows, research assistants, lecturers at: under-graduate medical schools, postgraduate medical schools or schools of health (you might do a job in a specific post and be able to work for higher degree in parallel[8]).
2 Special schemes such as LATS (London Academic Training Scheme) with a two-year salaried post that includes a day of protected educational sessions; or the Associate Physician Scheme, North West region based in Liverpool.
3 Training fellowships, e.g. RCGP research fellowship or NHS regional training fellowships, in conjunction with a super-visory academic unit. Post-holders continue in service posts with protected time for research and a higher degree attached to an academic unit, with variable amounts of supervision.
4 Register for a higher degree (M Phil, PhD, MD) while con-tinuing in your service post and gain an academic appoint-ment when you have obtained your qualification.

5 Join a Research Network of an academic unit, participating in data collection and/or the analysis stage of the research project.
6 Participate in teaching medical students in the community as part of a university programme.
7 Join a research general practice. These are few and far between. Some receive regional funding for protected time and infrastructure.[9]

*Success in the academic community is judged by*:

▶ numbers and quality (journal of publication) of peer-reviewed publications
▶ numbers, sources, magnitude of research grants gained
▶ numbers of students supervised for M Phil and MD/PhD gaining qualification
▶ national and international recognition – as demonstrated by presentations at conferences, being a member of peer review bodies or expert committees, respected positions, scholarly work.

*Career ladder*
You might specialise in research, education, health service management, health economics or a mix of these. Use your experience and/or qualifications for climbing the academic career ladder as a senior lecturer, then reader, and finally a professor in departments/units of:

▶ general practice
▶ primary care
▶ schools of health
▶ centres for health service management.

*Qualifications*:
M Phil: usually two to three years part-time, supervised, research-based degree; equivalent to two or three good publications in a peer-reviewed journal. You might undertake an accredited research methods course or learn research methods more informally.
MD (or DM) (doctorate): usually five or six years part-time, unsupervised-research-based degree. Usually gained from the

university in which candidate graduated, or a university in which the candidate holds a post.

PhD: usually five or six years part-time/three years full-time, supervised, research-based degree.

Both an MD and PhD involve undertaking original research that makes a significant contribution to the knowledge base.

---

**Pros and cons of an academic career**

*Plus points*:

- finding an answer to your research question can be exciting
- following a line of enquiry often takes you into new situations, meeting different people from those in your normal routine
- can be a ticket to international travel
- undertaking research teaches you to challenge received wisdom in your everyday life
- provides variety to your everyday work
- time taken can be flexible to fit in with your service work.

*Minus points*:[8–10]

- often less pay than in a service post
- opportunities not always advertised; levels of departmental support are variable
- academic doctors have a lower status than service doctors in some circles
- small numbers of posts, limited opportunities
- service work can limit time for academic research and education work
- no merit awards for senior GP academics
- NHS superannuation scheme not open to medical academics employed as a non-NHS university appointment
- registration for a higher qualification can seem expensive, especially if it takes many years to complete the degree because of the conflicting commitments of service work.

Association of Medical Research Charities, 29–35 Farringdon Road, London EC1 3JB.

Training Awards Groups, Medical Research Council, 20 Park Crescent, London W1N 4AL.

Department of Medical Education, School of Health, Staffordshire University, Blackheath Lane, Stafford ST18 0AD.

RN is 35 years old and has worked in academic primary care for five years. After vocational training he successfully applied for a two-year, full-time Research Training Fellowship funded by the (then) Regional Health Authority. During this time he completed the bulk of the work towards a PhD, began to publish, taught undergraduates and postgraduates, and maintained a limited clinical commitment in an honorary capacity at a local practice.

After the Fellowship he was appointed as a clinical lecturer in primary care, with responsibility for developing and running a primary care research network. At the same time he was appointed as a part-time principal at a local practice. His time is currently divided between research (both continuing his own programme of research, collaborating with and supervising others), teaching and service general practice.

'After house jobs I did various SHO posts around the country, having little idea of my ultimate career direction. Then I did a vocational training scheme to gave me some job security, I wanted to know where I would be. The course organiser heard about the research fellowship and passed it on to me. I think people thought it was a bit strange to be going into academic work and were a bit wary of me, but I had lots of informal careers advice on the way – I think I was lucky to meet the right people.'

## The armed forces

The Defence Medical Services recruit officers for all three services from fully qualified doctors who serve as short-service commissioned medical officers. Candidates under 40 years old who have served two years can then apply to convert to a regular commission. A limited number of cadetships are offered to medical students.

The same three-day selection process is followed as for all officers. Having joined the forces, medical students and junior doctors train in the same hospitals as civilians with an extra three months in military medicine and surgery and serve a minimum of six years.

General practice vocational training schemes at 23 of the 50 worldwide practices are inspected and approved by the JCPTGP. Not all disciplines are represented – geriatrics is a notable omission. Army public health (which includes family health and resource management) and occupational medicine (which includes aviation medicine) are recognised specialties.

Basic fitness training, military and service duties are included and even on leaving the services, personnel can be called up in times of war.

Job description

1 Medical care of forces personnel at home and around the world.
2 Care of civilian patients local to military hospitals.
3 Organisation and administration of field hospitals during active service.

Special characteristics:

- leadership
- confidence
- initiative
- sociability
- ability to make decisions under pressure
- tolerance of change often at short notice (the job can disrupt family life).

In addition doctors can work as civilian medical officers (CMO). Advertisements are placed in the *BMJ* from time to time and might specify an overseas location. These doctors provide general medical services to service personnel and their families without joining the services themselves. Posts are full time but often for a limited duration. A certificate from the JCPTGP is required just as for general practice.

Col. (retd) Tony Williams, Defence Medical Services, Officer Recruiting (RAMC), Keogh Barracks, Ash Vale, Aldershot, Hampshire GU12 5RQ. *Tel*: 01252 324431.

Director Medical Personnel, Personnel and Training, Room G76, RAF Innsworth, Gloucester GL3 1WZ. *Tel*: 01452 712612 (ex 5839).

Dean of Naval Medicine, Monckton House, Institute of Naval Medicine, Alverstoke, Gosport, Hampshire PO12 2DL. *Tel*: 01795 768000.

HQTA Army Medical Services (CMPs), Napier House, The Castle, Chester CH1 2YZ. *Tel*: 01244 352412.

TA now works as a GP in a group practice in a small market town, but she started her GP career in the air force. After completing her pre-registration house jobs in district general hospitals, she did her GP training with the Royal Air Force.

'I enjoyed my stint with the RAF immensely, but service life and young families don't mix well so that's why I left in the end. My training posts and later GP posts with the RAF were all sited at bases in England. I obtained a certificate of aviation medicine and another on radiation protection while with the RAF. My GP training posts with the RAF allowed me to develop my interests in orthopaedic medicine as well as doing more traditional posts such as obstetrics and gynaecology. Military experience in itself is useful; running a detachment to Africa certainly hones your 'people management' skills, which

I found to be a positive employment skill after I left. I have done GP locum work in military practices since leaving the RAF and would recommend a short spell to any GP who hasn't yet decided to settle down.'

## Forensic medicine

This is a collective term for a field that includes a number of posts, both part time and full time.

### Forensic physicians

Known as police surgeons, or forensic medical examiners in London, these are almost all GPs with a part-time contract with a police force. Some have the Diploma in Medical Jurisprudence of the Worshipful Society of Apothecaries (DMJ). Their duty is to examine and provide medical opinions on victims of assault, sexual offenders and drunk drivers. They are often called to certify deaths of unidentified bodies.

### Coroners

There are not many doctors who are coroners and most of them hold joint qualifications in law. Some GPs are coroners or deputies but recent regulations have recommended that only lawyers be appointed.

### Forensic pathology

Training posts are in university departments following general pathology training. Although they can also start out with part 1 of the DMJ, the second part is a specialist pathologist route. MRCPath (Forensic) is a highly specialised qualification; 48 post-holders are on the Home Office register and are called on to perform autopsies on major cases.

## Prison doctor

General medical services for prisoners is provided by 150 full-time and 100 part-time Home Office-employed prison doctors; some are visiting GPs. Forensic psychiatrists also visit prisoners with mental illness but they are mostly employed by the NHS. A diploma in prison medicine is offered jointly by the RCGP, RCP and RCPsych. This is a two-year modular course, each module taking a week full time, with six modules per year.

## Expert witness

Both defence and prosecuting lawyers call on expert medical advice from doctors not involved in their case, from time to time. Doctors called as witnesses for a case in which they have been involved are known as a 'professional witnesses'. The role of the 'expert witness' is to provide independent, objective and unbiased opinion on the facts of a case. Expert witnesses usually have considerable medical experience and knowledge of the medico-legal process and particular subjects. The 'Expert Witness Institute' offers skills training and courses on report writing.

Directorate of Health Care for Prisoners, Cleland House, Page Street, London SW1P 4LN. *Tel*: 020 7217 6497.

Association of Police Surgeons, 18a Mount Parade, Harrogate HG1 1BX. *Tel*: 01423 509 727.

Expert Witness Institute, 11 Haymarket, London SW1Y 4BP. *Tel*: 020 7930 7878.

GH is a GP and police surgeon

'We applied as a practice to become the police surgeons in our town when a circular came round from the police station. I have got the DMJ, but many don't have it. Whoever is on call for the day is also on call for the police and calls average about 30 per month.

Usual calls are to assess fitness to be detained, often if prisoners are on drugs or have ongoing medical conditions, especially suspected mental illnesses. We treat those injured during arrests or who have been assaulted, including police officers. We take blood for alcohol levels from those on the borderline of failing the breath test. Cot deaths and deaths in suspicious circumstances are also our responsibility but we only have to confirm death, the rest being up to a pathologist.

The worst event to which I have been called was to see a young lad who had fallen asleep on the railway line; but usually it is nothing as dreadful as that. The police are very protective of you in those circumstances. It is much worse for them because they have to go through the pockets of the corpse while we just have to confirm death.

There is a nationally agreed pay-scale but you can negotiate your own depending on specific local circumstances. If you are prepared to get up at night it is very well paid for what you actually do.'

## Medical defence organisations

The total number of doctors in the three main defence organisations is only around 30 so new jobs are few and far between and competition is fierce. New applicants will have at least six years of experience in a clinical field such as general practice or O&G. The Medical Protection Society requires doctors to undertake legal training and all doctors have a higher medical qualification such as the FRCS.

Regular in-house training programmes exist in civil law, ethics and NHS regulations.

Job description

▶ Assist and advise doctors in dealing with complaints, inquests, disciplinary hearings, criminal allegations and with the media.

- ▶ Written advice on ethical and legal matters.
- ▶ Participation in 24-hour telephone advice rota.
- ▶ Teaching and lecturing on risk management.

Special characteristics:

- ▶ objectivity
- ▶ maturity
- ▶ experience
- ▶ excellent communication skills
- ▶ good team player.

Medical Protection Society, Granary Wharf House, Leeds LS11 5PY. *Tel*: 0113 243 6436.

The Medical Defence Union, 192 Altrincham Road, Manchester M22 4RZ. *Tel*: 0161 428 1234.

Medical and Dental Defence, Union of Scotland, McIntosh House, 120 Blythwood Street, Glasgow G2 4EA. *Tel*: 0141 221 5858.

PD was originally a GP before he became an adviser to a medical defence organisation.

'As junior hospital doctors a great friend and I would from time to time discuss our futures. He was certain that he would not spend his entire career in one discipline, but after 20 years in a specialty would go into general practice. I took the view that it would not be possible to change a career after so long. We would be set in our ways, not relish the retraining, relocation and probable loss of seniority.

However, after 18 years working happily in general practice I saw an advertisement for a position with a medical defence organisation. The partnership I worked in was very progressive and I enjoyed being a trainer, but I was fired with enthusiasm at the prospect of a new challenge and a complete change of direction. I was fortunate since the opportunity arose at a time when it was possible to move and not disrupt my children's education, and even more fortunate to be appointed.

For the last ten years I have been assisting doctors with their medico-legal problems arising out of patient care. The organisation gave me excellent training in law and medical ethics applicable to the work, which is very diverse. It includes a large amount of telephone advice concerning problems as they happen, to discuss the options and possible ways forward. However, it is the direct personal contact helping members with their problems that I enjoy most, liaising where necessary with legal advisers and medical experts. I find it fascinating work.

My fellow house officer continues very successfully in his consultant post.'

## Overseas work

European directive 93/16/EEC provides for the mutual recognition by all member states of the medical qualifications of those doctors who are citizens of a member state and whose basic training was in a member state. Bureaucracy can be considerable and the language barrier puts most British doctors off. British-based embassies or High Commissions will be able to advise.

Of the 16% of doctors who leave the NHS per annum, most go overseas to work in Australia or New Zealand, developing countries or disaster areas. Registration with the local equivalent of the GMC will be required and in some countries (such as the USA and Canada) that means a qualifying examination.

Most charity work involves a drop in income and loss of job security. Some NHS trusts have agreements with Voluntary Services Overseas (VSO) that make it easier for doctors to take a sabbatical or temporary release with the knowledge that their job may be available to them on return. The BMA and the Royal Colleges are in favour of recognising VSO work as part of training. National insurance and pension contributions will be paid by VSO throughout the contract, but remuneration is consistent with the charitable status. Married doctors with families are rarely (if ever) accepted.

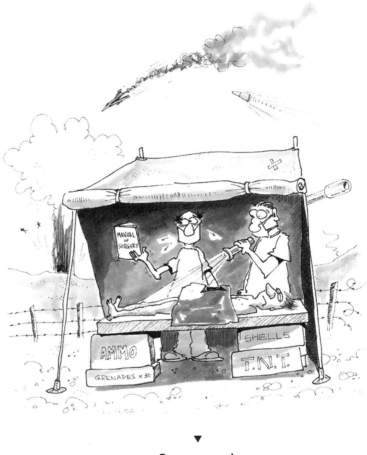

▼
**Overseas work**

Aid organisations hold a register of doctors prepared to fly out as required in times of war or natural disaster. Work like this can be challenging and rewarding but is complex to arrange and fraught with potential difficulties. The international department of the BMA should be able to advise about most of these matters, especially conditions of service overseas.

Medical Emergency Relief International (Merlin), 1A Rede Place, Chepstow Place, London W2 4TU. *Tel*: 020 7487 2505.

International Health Exchange, 8–10 Dryden Street, London WC2E 9NA. *Tel*: 020 7836 5833.

VSO Enquiries Unit, 317 Putney Bridge Road, London SW15 2PN. *Tel*: 020 8780 2266.

HR is a GP who spent five years in South Africa as medical officer in a Catholic mission hospital. His first big shock was being asked to provide a certificate of good standing from the GMC that there were no disciplinary hearings pending!

'I needed to register with the South African Medical Council, but the organisation I went with took care of most of that. Although there are plenty of South African doctors the area where I was is an under-served area so they were desperate for someone with any experience at all. I would say though that you are better off if you have at least five years under your belt, because you might end up being the only doctor out there. I had the Diploma in Anaesthetics, which was very useful not just for operating but as an introduction to the only type of life support that was really possible – pretty basic. You need an enormous amount of energy, the work can be unlimited and you have to be well-motivated. We ran a sort of health visitor training programme for the local women that was very worthwhile; really just about immunisation, nutrition and rehydration therapy.

I will never forget the things I saw and some of the people I met. I think the experience has changed me and not always for the better! I see middle-class mothers worried about their perfectly well children and I have to summon up all my reserves to be sympathetic.'

# Parallel tracks: what are the jobs that might contribute to a portfolio career?

*Community health*

This is an area of primary care where much work is sessional and hours are flexible. It is largely concerned with the health of children and women. There have been some changes to the career structure over the past few years that mean there is sometimes an on-call commitment as posts are linked to hospital rotations and rotas, but it is still much more suitable for those with other commitments, such as caring for a young family.

Family planning and reproductive health is now organised by the Faculty of that name at the Royal College of Obstetricians and Gynaecologists. Community paediatrics is organised by the Royal College of Paediatrics and Child Health. Both fields are developing higher specialist training programmes and career structures.

Child health surveillance is now a requirement for all practices and for the MRCGP. Child development clinics and clinics for those children with special needs can be staffed by specialists or GPs with a special interest. Community health is now becoming consultant-led and new appointments are as staff grades (formally Clinical Medical Officers) and associate specialists (SCMOs).

Most contraception in this country is provided in general practice and some GPs also work in family planning clinics. Community gynaecologists are increasing in number and these two types of doctor often work side by side offering services in pyschosexual counselling, GU medicine and health education.

Faculty of Family Planning and Reproductive Healthcare, 27 Sussex Place, Regent's Park, London NW1 4RG. *Tel*: 020 7723 3175.

Royal College of Paediatrics and Child Health, 50 Hallam Street, London W1N 6DE. *Tel*: 020 7307 5600.

JW finished general practice training but then moved to a new area because her husband changed jobs. She had two small children and when she saw an advertisement for sessional family planning doctors she found the hours very suitable. She applied, and was accepted on, to a bank of doctors who could be called on to staff family planning clinics as and when needed. Other doctors sharing the rota were clinical medical officers, a higher specialist trainee in community gynaecology and GPs, as well as one part-time A&E trainee.

'I had the old family planning certificate which I converted to the Diploma of the Faculty of Family Planning when it was set up. It is not as well paid as sessions in general practice, about £50 for a two-hour session that sometimes extends to three hours, but the hours and the flexibility mean that you can work just when it suits you. It can be organised around family life. The work is varied and interesting. We do the usual coil fitting and pill prescriptions but also counselling about HIV/AIDS and termination of pregnancy and sexual health.

I am an assistant in general practice now but I still do family planning sessions. There is always a need for doctors, even though there is now a higher specialist training pathway for consultants in family planning, because the throughput of doctors is so rapid and they tend to come and go.'

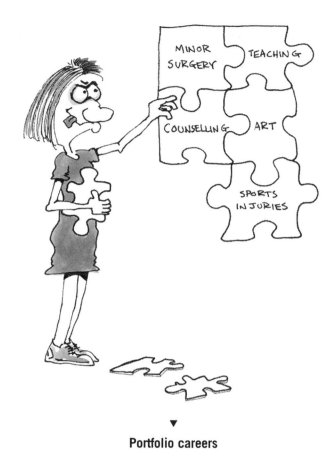

**Portfolio careers**

## Complementary medicine

It is possible to earn a living solely in private practice, especially for those holding joint medical and alternative qualifications, a rare combination. Medical practitioners will be in competition with lay practitioners and will need business and marketing skills to be successful. A range of SHO posts or training in general practice will be more likely to equip you to set up a private clinic than experience of a single specialty.

Many complementary therapies are also available on the NHS and some doctors combine mainstream medicine with an interest or expertise in a complementary therapy. Acupuncture,

homeopathy and hypnotherapy can be combined with ortho-
dox medicine and many courses exist, some of which lead to
national accreditation.

British Medical Acupuncture Society, Acupuncture Society,
Newton Lane, Whitley, Warrington, Cheshire WA4 4JA.
*Tel*: 01925 730727.

Royal London Homeopathic Hospital, Great Ormond Street,
London W1. *Tel*: 020 7837 8833.

British Medical and Dental Hypnosis Society, 17 Keppell
View Road, Kimberworth, Rotherham, South Yorks S61 2AR.
*Tel*: 01709 554558.

Anglo-European College of Chiropractic, 13–15 Parkwood
Road, Boscombe, Bournemouth, Dorset BH5 2DF. *Tel*:
01202 436200.

JS is a principal in general practice who offers his patients
acupuncture alongside conventional medicine. Encouraged by
colleagues who reported good results with difficult-to-treat
conditions such as low back pain and tennis elbow, he went
on a course run by the British Medical Acupuncture Society
(the BMAS). Initially sceptical, he was won over by patients'
feedback.

'There are patients who either cannot take anti-inflammatory
medication or who would rather not take tablets and acupuncture gives us another option. The thing is that it actually
does work. It's a bit like cricket though, you have to suspend
your disbelief. Acupuncturists use funny words and for a
doctor that can be difficult since we have a certain map of the
body. The BMAS course is run by doctors for doctors. They
have a good certification procedure and rigorous training and
the induction is very short so you can start practising and
seeing results quickly. The course is over two weekends about
a month apart so you put into practice what you have learnt
and then build on that.

Patients are seen in normal surgery. I put the needles in then the patient waits in a separate room while I move on to the next appointment. I have only forgotten to go back twice!'

## Postgraduate general practice education

This is one of the most varied options open to GPs. All GP registrars are trained in practices where one or more of the partners is a trainer. Each deanery is responsible for training the trainers and inspecting training practices. The trainer is the most important person involved in GP training. He or she has a one-to-one relationship with the GP registrar for up to a year. The trainer acts as an educational supervisor and mentor supporting the registrar through the summative assessment process and helping in preparation for the Membership of the Royal College of General Practitioners (MRCGP) examination. The trainer is paid an allowance to support these activities.

Vocational training day-release schemes are run by course organisers who may also have a responsibility for SHO posts approved for general practice training. GP tutors plan and organise the continuing professional education for GPs in each district, often based in the local hospital postgraduate centre. These posts can be very rewarding, but are hard work and the time taken to do them well outstrips the money nominally paid to cover them. Many of those involved in general practice education are qualified in education over and above being trained as trainers. Certificates in medical education are available from certain universities and Teaching the Teacher basic skills courses are run by many postgraduate deans.

After gaining experience as a course organiser or GP tutor it is possible to become an associate director or director of post-graduate GP education (DPGPE). These important positions involve setting and monitoring standards of GP education in the deanery and contributing to strategic development of GP training nationally.

MF is one of three course organisers who runs a local vocational training scheme. He started by becoming the GP trainer in his practice when the previous trainer retired and he had been a GP principal for five years. He really enjoyed the GP trainer courses and workshops, so that when there was a vacancy as a GP course organiser he applied for the two half-days a week post. His partners are happy to let him go as he pays his salary into the practice account which enables the practice to employ a GP working on the retainer scheme in his place.

'I love teaching the GP registrars and young hospital doctors. Many of them have become quite cynical as a result of gruelling hospital posts where they feel their skills and contribution have not been valued as they should. We help them learn from their experiences. I am registered for a Masters in Education at a local university to help me develop my teaching skills. I'm learning to try out different methods of teaching and am setting objectives and evaluating our sessions much more effectively. I have been a course organiser for five years and my post is about to come up for renewal when I'll have to re-apply for my job. I want to remain a course organiser if possible as I enjoy the contact with young doctors so much.'

## Journalism

There are two routes to medical journalism: freelance and by attachment to specialist medical journals, newspapers or radio and television. The former is more common and both are hard work and very competitive. Medical journalists are better paid than their lay counterparts.

Those with a flair for the written word can try sending off articles to the press, especially the weekly medical magazines, although unsolicited copy is less commonly accepted than that commissioned from well-known medical personalities. Brevity, reliability, keeping to agreed deadlines and succinct use of language are essential characteristics.

There is a professional organisation for medical journalists and a Medical Writers Association; membership of either will forge good contacts. The *BMJ* offers a one-year registrar post in medical journalism open to doctors with 3–5 years' clinical experience and the *BMA News Review* offers one-day introductory courses. An ex-editor of the *News Review*, Tim Albert, now runs a consultancy in medical communication organising good training in writing skills.

Medical Journalists Association, 2 St Georges Road, Kingston upon Thames, Surrey KT2 6DN. *Tel*: 020 8549 1019.

National Union of Journalists, Acorn House, 314 Gray's Inn Road, London WC1X 8DP. *Tel*: 020 7278 7916.

GP Writers Association, 633 Liverpool Road, Southport, Merseyside PR8 3NG. *Tel*: 01704 577 839.

Tim Albert Training. *Tel*: 01306 877993; *E-mail*: tatraining @compuserve.com

RR is a GP whose work is often published in medical weeklies. She started by sending in ideas for an article about GPs' hobbies to the editor of a well-known GP newspaper because a friend had had an article accepted previously. That first article led to commissions for other articles and she quickly built up a reputation for writing on a wide variety of topics in many other newspapers and journals for the medical, nursing and lay press.

'It's an amazing feeling to get your first article accepted. It was difficult to believe that other people would find it worthwhile to read what I had written. Being published has given me increased confidence and maintained my self-esteem. Being a writer gives you a lot of energy for everyday life as you think deeply about the issues and start to be more challenging and enjoy your own powers of observation. I carry a notebook around in my handbag, and often jot down thoughts for new articles or insights that I might want to relay in my writing. It is relatively good pay; each newspaper or journal has a standard rate per word length. Over the years I was a full-time GP I earned about 10% of my income from writing, but that was at the expense of a lot of my time at home being spent on writing. Now I write books and earn much less from writing them than commissioned articles.'

## Management

MBA courses are available in many universities and offer suitable training for entry for doctors into management in the NHS. Trust management structure, PCGs, health authorities, Department of Health or NHS Executive are all places where a management-trained doctor can make a substantial contribution. The private sector and work outside the NHS are also options.

British Association of Medical Managers, Barnes Hospital, Kingsway, Cheadle, Cheshire SK8 2NY. *Tel*: 0161 491 4229.

JM is a partner in general practice who did a part-time MBA, initially for the challenge of something a bit different. Realising how many doors it opened for her after that, she responded to an advertisement for a part-time primary care adviser for the health authority.

'I think we need more real-life GPs in positions like this in the health authority if the primary care-led NHS is going to be anything more than just a government sound bite. Most of the paperwork I receive is total gobbledygook, but if it seems like that to me then it will be viewed like that by those on PCG boards too. I can inject some realism and common sense into the content and language of documents. You have to have understanding partners though. Like everything else, the work expands into the time available to do it and there is never enough time in the week to fit it all in.'

## Medical advisers

Occasionally, unstructured positions come up in a variety of organisations as advisers, for example to first-aid organisations such as the Red Cross, health authorities and statutory bodies such as the Human Fertilisation and Embryology Authority. These are usually sessional and sometimes unpaid.

Medical advisers of health authorities were originally pre-retirement GPs who acted as the liaison between the health authority and GPs in an area. They oversee aspects such as child health surveillance, minor surgery and health promotion, and interpret and advise on the Red Book, the terms and conditions of service in general practice.

The Department of Social Security employs many medical advisers, typically as examining officers for the Benefits Agency. Medicals for eligibility for the Disability Living Allowance are carried out by doctors who have had a four-day training course followed by a written assessment of knowledge and supervised sessions with a trainer.

The Independent Tribunal Service panels hear appeals about social security, vaccine damage, disability appeals and child support issues. The membership is varied but the doctors on the panels have an induction course and members have to observe appeals before they are allowed to become full panel members. Fees are paid on an hourly and sessional basis.

Chief Medical Officer, Benefits Agency (see local telephone directory).

Independent Tribunal Service (Midlands), *Tel*: 0121 643 6464.

AW is a medical adviser with a health authority. Having originally trained as a pharmacist, he was drawn to medicine for the hands-on involvement with patients. After some time as a GP principal, however, he felt that he could make more of a contribution in public health medicine. He had passed the MRCGP and was able to enter into higher specialist training which culminated in MFPHM. After one year as a consultant in public health medicine he was offered the job with the health authority. Four years later he has now returned to general practice as a principal.

'I felt as though I was trying to hold back the tide when I was a GP. I was looking onwards to the next 35 years and really felt like doing something else before settling down to practice.

The job description tends to vary from one health authority to another. At the moment it is very much about primary care development and supporting primary care groups. There is no real training required – although it was handy to have the MFPHM, it certainly isn't a requirement. You need to be a principal with about 3–5 years in practice. Most health authorities are flexible about parallel sessions in general practice, in fact some clinical work is encouraged as a way of retaining credibility with GPs.'

## Medical politics

The local medical committee (LMC) is a representative body to which all GPs pay a statutory levy deducted at source and they may pay a voluntary levy as well. When a health authority wants to consult or negotiate with GPs it has traditionally done so through the LMC. There are statutory duties relating to the individual interests of GPs, and medico-political functions are mainly concerned with the collective interests of GPs as a group. Depending on local arrangements, non-principals and trainees can be represented and new members can volunteer to stand at election time. Dentists, optometrists and pharmacists also have local committees. The relationship of the LMC to PCGs and PCTs is still evolving.

D H-F has been a LMC member for several years. He feels he drifted into it when encouraged by a colleague, but has held different positions on the committee and subcommittee and is now chair.

'There are not exactly hundreds flocking to stand at election times and it does tend to be the same old people so there are always opportunities for new blood to get involved. There are geographical constituencies and about 12 of us represent around 250 GPs. Primarily we exist to represent and support GPs and we are the only body that is run solely by GPs for GPs. We try to ensure that GMS activities are protected, supported and not threatened.

We work in a healthy atmosphere of "evidence-based cynicism". You definitely need to enjoy it because it can be time-consuming. I am paid for one session a week, but do at least one more. It is very different from sitting in surgery and gives a perspective on medicine in its broadest sense. You meet a lot of people you would not otherwise come across and that can be quite an eye-opener. Because we are elected by GPs, we can enter into rigorous discussions with the powers-that-be without worrying about our positions or losing our jobs.'

MC is a member of a PCG Board.

'No one knows how this is all going to work out yet, but it is very exciting to be involved at the cutting edge of the new NHS. I think people see us as the implementers of government policy and I know that a lot of people feel that that policy has been made up on a whim. But it is more than that. We can influence local issues and the health authority really needs to work with us if it is truly to be a primary care-led service.

The remuneration is meagre because there is far more to do than time allowed to do it in. Committee meetings tend to expand as the heath authority expects unlimited advice and information. The opportunity to understand more about social services has been one of the best aspects of the job.'

## Sports and exercise medicine

Doctors in these posts are often athletic themselves with an interest in sport. There are at least three types of sports doctor, all mostly part-time posts and usually undertaken by GPs.

## Sports injury clinics

Usually for those patients involved in sport recreationally. GPs with a Diploma in sports medicine often run these either in practice or in hospitals in conjunction with the physiotherapy department and sometimes an interested orthopaedic surgeon. There are some private sports injuries clinics, mostly in London.

## Professional club doctor

These are often attached to athletic or football clubs representing much greater levels of sporting expertise and requiring concomitant levels of experience from the doctors. Pay is usually sessional, sometimes with a retainer for more formal arrangements.

## Full-time professional athletics physician

These are very uncommon posts. An MSc in sports medicine is available at Nottingham University for this level of involvement. Terms and conditions of service vary between posts and there are no set levels for fees. A knowledge of drugs in sport, nutrition and travel problems is important.

The British Association of Sport and Medicine runs short courses for those interested in sports medicine, and the National Sports Medicine Institute organises three-year, part-time studies. The Society of Apothecaries of London offers a Diploma course. The International Council offers a range of services including professional insurance and legal advice.

British Association of Sport and Medicine, c/o National Sports Medicine Institute, Medical College St Bart's Hospital, Charterhouse Square, London EC1M 6BQ. *Tel*: 020 7251 0583.

International Institute of Sports Therapy, 46 Aldwick Road, Bognor Regis PO21 2PN. *Tel*: 01243 842 064.

International Council of Health, Fitness and Sports Therapists, 38a Portsmouth Road, Woolston, Southampton SO2 9AD. *Tel*: 01703 422 695.

CW is a GP and club doctor for a second division professional football club.

'We were approached as a practice a few years ago when the medical officer on the board retired. They needed a new doctor because it is a pre-requisite of the Football Association for matches where the crowd will number more than 5000. The match can't go ahead without a doctor. In fact there should be two, one for the crowd and one for the players.

So we take it in turns. We attend all matches and we do a round at the club every Tuesday for the walking wounded. We are also available for some of the players to come to surgery. The work is mainly dealing with inter-current illnesses in the players, psychological complaints as well as musculo-skeletal injuries. Two of us have a diploma in sports medicine. Since the Hillsborough disaster all those responsible for the crowd have to go on triage training as well, just in case.

It's quite a commitment but relatively easy since we do it as a practice. You rarely have to deal with fractures from flying tackles but it's interesting and varied and you do get to see some good games occasionally!'

# References

1  Whitehouse AB (1999) *Postgraduate Medical and Dental Education Careers Information pack*. West Midlands Deanery, Birmingham.

2  Wilkinson D (1999) Anaesthesia. *BMJ Classified, Career Focus*. **27 March**: 2–3.

3 Sulkin T (1999) Clinical radiology. *BMJ Classified, Career Focus*. **27 March**: 2–3.

4 Williams N (1999) Training in occupational medicine. *Update*. **20 May**: 970–2.

5 Lloyd-Williams M (1999) Palliative medicine. *BMJ Classified, Career Focus*. **2 July**: 2–3.

6 Marshall W (1998) Pathology. *BMJ Classified, Career Focus*. **10 Oct**: 2–3.

7 Goldin J (1999) Child and adolescent psychiatry. *BMJ Classified, Career Focus*. **17 July**: 2–3.

8 Lester H, Carter Y, Dassu D *et al.* (1998) Survey of research activity, training needs, departmental support, and career intentions of junior academic general practitioners. *Br J Gen Pract*. **48**: 1322–6.

9 Pereira Gray D (Chairman) (1996) *Developing Primary Care. The academic contribution*. RCGP, London.

10 Richards R and Kinmouth AL (eds) (1997) *Clinical Academic Careers: report of an independent task force*. Committee of Vice-Chancellors and Principals, London.

# CHAPTER 6

# What now? Making the jump

Having considered all your options you may find yourself contemplating applying for a new job. Whether it is a complete career change or an extra job, much of the process of application is similar. For most posts, selection will be made by an appointments committee on the basis of an application form (including a curriculum vitae), references and interview with or without a presentation, although these methods have been criticised.[1,2]

Each post and appointments committee will be different so there are no hard and fast rules. In general practice, it is still common for spouses to be invited to the so-called 'trial by sherry'. Try to maintain a sense of humour throughout, which is not always easy.

Popular advice is not to antagonise interview panels by questioning or even arguing a point. But consider how you will fit into an organisation that does not think in a similar way to you. The interview may be the first time you realise that you are incompatible. Be honest with yourself and the interview panel. It is especially important that you are all compatible in general practice as these will be your business partners.

Some of the points below should be relevant to your situation; not all will be applicable for all interviews.

## Your CV

Your curriculum vitae (CV) is your shop window. It has to be good enough to get you that interview so that your undoubted qualities have an opportunity to shine through. Pay attention to the following points:

1 A poorly organised CV may be interpreted as evidence of poor communication skills. Think carefully about layout. Make sure that your strengths are clearly presented.
2 Do not go into too much detail about your earlier years, but make sure all dates are correct and there are no gaps to account for. If you have had a career break be prepared to justify it.
3 Tailor your CV for each application. Identify important information in the advertisement and the person specification and draw the attention of the people short-listing to your suitability by summarising your key strengths on a front page.
4 Consider a competency-based CV. Explain how it is that you are competent for the job you have applied for. This does not concentrate on what posts you have held, but what you have achieved. So it might state, for example, that you learnt basic surgical principles during your surgical house job, performed operations X, Y and Z unassisted in a casualty post, went on a minor surgery course and are now on the health authority list for minor surgery.
5 Resist the temptation to say 'please see CV' if an application form is required to be filled in.
6 Spelling mistakes are inexcusable with word-processed CVs. Get someone to proofread it for you for other errors. Consider asking a senior colleague for their comments.

Once short-listed you must be prepared to capitalise on your achievements. Increasingly candidates are asked to prepare a presentation on a given topic. This is your opportunity to give a slick demonstration of your communication, organisational and information technology skills.

# Preparing for the interview

1 Speak to the present incumbent if it is a hospital post and the key personnel in the department. For example, if an obstetric job involves ultrasound, speak to the radiographers. Consider meeting the chair of the local PCG or PCT. Try to find out what the local issues are for the trust and the department.

2 In general practice, there is much to be revealed by visiting the practice during surgery hours. Is the waiting room full? Are the receptionists flustered? Perhaps you could engage a patient in conversation and speak to the practice manager. Look at the standard of maintenance, does a tatty building mean tatty organisation too?

3 Ask for a copy of the annual report or practice accounts. It will help you to gauge the size and strength of the organisation, as well as give you ammunition to ask intelligent questions. Is there a practice development plan with an associated educational plan?

4 Decide why you want the post, what you want from the post and what compromises you can make.

5 Consider a visit to a clinic or surgery to get a feel for the work of the department or practice. The BMA has produced guidelines for observers of clinical practice which should be adhered to.[3]

6 Plan some questions that show your interests, what are the research opportunities like for example, or the continuing medical education facilities? What do they think about the postgraduate centre library?

7 Don't assume they can remember the details in your CV – or have read it even.

8 Consider preparing a short aide-mémoire handout that you can leave behind, so that they can remember which candidate you were. Nothing too ostentatious though.

# The big day

By the time you get called for an interview, the panel have already seen something in your application that makes them want to take a look. Remember this if you think you are starting to flounder. The better prepared you are the less likely it is that someone can bowl you a 'googly'. The interview is designed to test your reactions under stress to a certain extent, often the interviewer is more interested in the way you handle a question than the content of what you say.

1 Dress to impress. Old-fashioned advice? You are trying to sell yourself as competent and capable. Having said that, be yourself and express your personality, you must feel comfortable.

2 The first few questions will be designed to put you at your ease and settle the nerves. Make eye contact, smile and look interested. If you can remember the names of anybody as they are introduced to you that is a bonus. Avoid saying 'It is all there in my application form'. These are your starters-for-ten.

3 Some questions are predictable. Have answers for the following.
   - Why do you want to work here?
   - What are your strengths …
   - … and weaknesses? If they ask this try to think of a weakness that you have adjusted, for example 'I'm not very good at time management, but I am learning to delegate more'.
   - What skills will you bring to the team?

4 Be up to date with current medical issues. Read the journals, have a view.

5 Do not be put off by apparently biased questions, especially about gender issues. It is unlikely that the interviewer is really sexist, he or she may be testing your reactions. Sometimes humour helps.

6 Some questions can be unnerving if you do not know the answer. The best thing is to admit your ignorance but say

how you would go about finding out 'That is an interesting question', 'I would have to look that up/ask someone.'

7 Find the balance between thinking before you speak and thinking out loud if you are unsure about an answer. Interviewers may be interested in how you approach a question even if you do not know instantly what they are driving at. If you do put your foot in it, do not dig any deeper. It is okay to say 'Actually now I think about it, that's a daft answer' and have another stab at it.

8 Honesty and integrity show through. Do not try to second-guess the 'correct' answer. Politics are unlikely to be overtly discussed but issues such as rationing of healthcare, private medicine, how the lottery money should be spent, may be. Say what you think and try to justify it.

9 Some interviewers specialise in unusual questions, especially in general practice. Have a think about the following questions:
   ▶ What book are you reading at the moment?
   ▶ Which famous people, past or present, would you like to invite to dinner?
   ▶ Who was more important: Florence Nightingale or Marie Curie?
   ▶ If you were stuck in a lift with the Health Minister, what would you say?

## The presentation

Think of a presentation as an opportunity not a threat, as a challenge rather than a problem. Try and see it from the interviewers' perspectives. It is a very boring task to interview half a dozen people who may be very similarly qualified on paper. In a presentation, you are in control and you can make sure the panel sees your strengths. The Institute of Management has published many books that can help with this type of task.[4]

1 Your talk should be concise and well-prepared. Make sure that you understand the task and stick to it.

2 Time yourself and keep to the time limit. It is surprising how long those short notes you wrote can last. (Conversely, you may find you deliver the talk much faster on the day.)

3 Try to make the presentation interesting with appropriate use of visual aids. Only use technology that you are familiar with; today is not the day to learn about PowerPoint presentations if you have never done that before.

4 A few well-designed overheads delivered slowly with a strong message will be more effective than an all-singing, all-dancing presentation, even if the latter is more eye-catching. It will also be less easy for you to make a mistake.

5 Practise presenting out loud at home.

6 Give yourself plenty of time to arrive and set up.

## Your golden opportunity

At the end of nearly every interview comes the question 'Is there anything you would like to ask us?' This should not be met merely with a sigh of relief that the interview is nearly over, but grasped with both hands as your opportunity both to show your enthusiasm for the post and to find out some more details.

1 You could ask about standards: e.g. do they do regular audit, is the department approved by the Royal Colleges for post-graduate training, how are notes kept, is it an electronic- or paper-based practice?

2 How is the workload shared and what are the outside commitments of those in the department or practice? Are consultants on lots of committees leaving the incoming doctor to do a disproportionate share of routine work? Or are the other colleagues' commitments prestigious to enhance practice/trust work? What proportion of their time do the consultants spend in private practice?

3 Is there a team approach or is there a sense of autocratic leadership? This can be a tricky area to uncover the truth.

A question such as 'Who makes the final decision if there is disagreement?' may be revealing.

4 What is the potential to maximise income either by private practice or outside jobs in general practice?

5 What is the availability of study leave? How are study leave and holidays organised? Are there restrictions on how many can be away at once?

6 What is the information technology infrastructure and support like?

7 Does the department or practice have links with others for support or educational activities?

# Referees

People usually think hard about who they will nominate as referees. It makes sense to choose someone whom you think will speak well of you. However, the influence a referee can have is often exaggerated.

The main reason for providing references is to ensure that there is objective confirmation of a candidate's history. A reference says more about the referee than the applicant. References should be used to confirm what has been discovered through the short-listing and interviewing process. While the qualitative information within a reference may be able to make a difference if two candidates are very close, they are the least important part of the application process. A poor reference is not much help to the candidate, but a good reference is not much help to the panel.

# References

1 Cook M (1998) Traditional ways of selecting medical staff. *BMJ Classified*. 7 **March**: 2–3.

2 Cook M (1998) New approaches to selecting medical staff. *BMJ Classified*. 14 **March**: 2–3.

3   British Medical Association (1999) *Work Observation Guidelines. Career progress of doctors committee*. British Medical Association, London.

4   Jay R (1995) *Effective Presentation*. The Institute of Management Foundation. Pitman, London.

# Further sources of information

## Books and information leaflets

*Medical careers: options and development*

Allen I (1994) *Doctors and Their Careers*. Policy Studies Institute, London.

Allen I (1998) *Any Room at the Top? A study of doctors and their careers*. Policy Studies Institute, London.

Anderson C (1996) *How to Organise a Careers Forum for General Practice*. University of Nottingham, Nottingham.

Anderson C and Turner R (1998) *Career Handbook for Medical Students*. University of Nottingham, Nottingham.

British Medical Association (1994) *Guidelines for Good Practice in the Recruitment and Selection of Doctors*. Career Progress of Doctors Committee, British Medical Association, London.

British Medical Association (1996) *Guidelines for the Provision of Careers Services for Doctors*. British Medical Association, London.

British Medical Association (1998) *Medical Careers: a general guide* (4e). British Medical Association, London.

British Medical Association (1998) *Doctors' Pay*. British Medical Association, London. (Describes pay structures and pay levels for various branches of the profession and other employed posts, such as police surgeon, armed forces doctors, deputising doctors.)

Calvert S and Urmston I (eds) (1998) *The Insider Guide to Medical Schools*. British Medical Journal, London.

Hall H, Dwyer D and Lewis T (eds) (1999) *The GP Training Handbook* (3e). Blackwell Science, London

Hopkins D (1999) *So ... You want to be a Doctor?* Kogan Page, London.

Iserson KV (1997) *Get into Medical School: a guide for the perplexed*. Galen Press, Tucson.

Johnson C, Forrest F and Hall C (1998) *Getting Ahead in Medicine*. BIOS Scientific Publishers, Oxford.

McKenna F and Pickersgill D (eds) (1995) *The GP's Guide to Professional and Private Work Outside the NHS*. Radcliffe Medical Press, Oxford.

Morrell J and Roberts A (1995) Make an application for flexible (part time) training. *BMJ*. **311**: 242–4.

NHS Executive (1996) *Making Your Choice in Medicine*. NHS Executive, London.

Norfolk Health Authority (1993) *Job Sharing in General Practice*. Human Resources Department, Norfolk Health Authority, Norfolk.

Petchey R, Williams J and Baker M (1996) *Junior Doctors, Medical Careers and General Practice*. University of Nottingham, Nottingham.

Richards P and Stockhill S (1997) *The New Learning Medicine*. BMJ Publishing, Plymouth.

Royal College of General Practitioners (1996) *Women General Practitioners*. RCGP Information Sheet No. 14. Royal College of General Practitioners, London.

Royal College of General Practitioners (1997) *Additional Career Options in General Practice*. RCGP Information Sheet No. 18. Royal College of General Practitioners, London.

Royal College of General Practitioners (1999) *Rural General Practice*. RCGP Information Sheet No 23. Royal College of General Practitioners, London.

Rushton J and Burnett J (1998) *Getting into Medical School*. Trotman, Surrey.

Ward C and Eccles S (1997) *So You Want to be a Brain Surgeon? A medical careers guide*. Oxford Medical Publications, Oxford.

Whitehouse AB (1999) *Careers Information Pack*. Postgraduate Medical and Dental Education, West Midlands Deanery, Birmingham.

Women in Medicine (1998) *Careers for Women in Medicine: planning and pitfalls*. Women in Medicine Collective, 21 Wallingford Avenue, London W10 6QA.

Women in Medicine. *Job-sharing and Part-time Work in General Practice* (booklet). Women in Medicine, 21 Wallingford Avenue, London W10 6QA.

## Career counselling

Ball B (1996) *Assessing Your Career: time for a change?* British Psychological Society, London.

Burnard P (1994) *Counselling Skills for Health Professionals*. Chapman and Hall, Cheltenham.

Hopson B and Scally M (1999) *Build Your Own Rainbow. A workbook for career and life management*. Management Books 2000, Chalford.

Nathan R and Hill L (1992) *Career Counselling*. Sage Publications, London.

Nelson-Jones R (1993) *You Can Help*. Cassell, London.

Nelson-Jones R (1996) *Practical Counselling and Helping Skills*. Cassell, London.

Reddy M (1987) *The Manager's Guide to Counselling at Work*. British Psychological Society/Routledge, London.

## Career development (general literature)

Booher D (1997) *Get Ahead, Stay Ahead! Learn the 70 most important career skills, traits and attitudes to: stay employed, get promoted, get a better job*. McGraw-Hill, London.

Eggert M (1999) *Perfect CV*. Arrow Business Books, London.

Francis D (1996) *Managing Your Own Successful Career*. Fontana, London.

Handy C (1995) *The Age of Unreason*. Arrow Business Books, London.

Kent S (1997) *Creating Your Own Career. Practical advice for graduates in a changing world*. Kogan Page, London.

Leider R (1994) *Life Skills: taking charge of your personal and professional growth*. Pfeiffer, London.

Nelson Bolles R (1996) *What Colour is Your Parachute? A practical manual for job hunters and career changers*. Ten Speed Press, California.

Schein E (1990) *Career Anchors: discovering your real needs*. Pfeiffer, Oxford.

Schein E (1990) *Career Anchors: trainer's manual*. Pfeiffer, Oxford.

### Personality types

Hanmer A (1993) *Introduction to Type and Careers*. Oxford Psychologists Press, Oxford.

Myers IB and Myers P (1995) *Gifts Differing: understanding personality types*. Davies Black Publishing, California.


**Writing skills**

Turner B (ed) (1999) *The Writer's Handbook*. Macmillan, London.


# Courses – examples

GP tutor Dr Ian Sidford in Redditch brings out an annual booklet describing part-time and distance-learning degrees, diploma, certificate, PGEA and other courses for medical practitioners in the UK. Contact Primary Care Department, University of Wolverhampton.

Ashridge development programmes for executives in management and organisation development. Ashridge Management College, Berkhamsted, Hertfordshire HP4 1NS. *E-mail*: info@ashridge.org.uk

Centre for Health Planning and Management, University of Keele. Run senior management programmes, the diploma in management for doctors, full- and part-time MBA (Health Executive) programme. Darwin Building, University of Keele, Keele, Staffs ST5 5BG. *Fax*: 01782 711737.

Diploma in Occupational Medicine. The Institute of Occupational Health at the University of Birmingham for the Diploma examination of the Faculty of Occupational Medicine. The Distance Learning Unit of the Centre for Occupational Health at the University of Manchester also runs a Diploma course, as do several other universities.

Health Services Management Centre, University of Birmingham. Runs leadership and management development programmes for senior managers and clinicians in the NHS as well as a range of targeted short courses. Park House, 40 Edgbaston Park Road, Birmingham B15 2RT. *Internet*: http://www.bham.ac.uk/hsmc/

Health Services Management Unit, University of Manchester. NHS management development programmes. Devonshire House, University Precinct Centre, Oxford Road, Manchester M13 9PL. *Fax*: 0161 273 5245.

Institute of Health and Care Development. Run career development programmes for mid-career NHS staff in England. IHCD, St Bartholomews Court, 18 Christmas Street, Bristol BS1 5BT. *Tel*: 0117 906 5500; *Internet*: http://www.ihcd.org.uk

King's Fund Management College. Programmes for general management, personal and professional development and leadership in the NHS. 11–13 Cavendish Square, London W1M 0AN. *Tel*: 020 7307 2400; *Internet*: http://www.kingsfund. org.uk

Open University Business School. Runs management development programmes. The Open University, Milton Keynes MK7 6AA. *Tel*: 01908 858437; *Fax*: 01908 858438; *Internet*: http://cehep.open.ac.uk

# Organisations or bodies providing careers advice or help

Association for the Study of Medical Education (ASME), ASME Office, 4th Floor, Hobart House, 80–82 Hanover Street, Edinburgh EH2 1EL. *Tel*: 0131 225 9111; *Fax*: 0131 225 9444; *E-mail*: info@asme.org.uk

British Association of Medical Managers (BAMM), Barnes Hospital, Kingsway, Cheadle, Cheshire SK8 2NY. *Fax*: 0161 491 4254. BAMM organises management and leadership development programmes, organises conferences and supports members.

British Medical Association, BMA House, Tavistock Square, London WC1H 0JP. *Tel*: 020 7387 4499. For details about national terms and conditions for doctors, and careers literature.

Careers Advice Service. Electronic, free and confidential careers advice on the doctors.net.uk website. All medical doctors in the UK with a GMC registration number (or provisional number) may seek advice. *Internet*: http://www.doctors.net.uk (access section on *Jobs*, and click on *Careers Advice*).

Career Track International. Seminars, audio and video tapes on management and leadership skills. Career Track International, Sunrise House, Sunrise Parkway, Linford Wood, Milton Keynes MK14 6YA. *Answerphone*: 01908 354101 (tapes), 01908 354000 (seminars); *Internet*: http://www.career track.com

Department for Education and Employment, Overseas Labour Service, W5 Moorfoot, Sheffield S1 4PQ. *Tel*: 0114 259 4074.

Executive Choice, the NHS Senior Career Development Service. Executive Choice, Dearden Management, Church Road, Redhill, Bristol BS18 7SG. *Tel*: 01934 863183; *Internet*: www. nhs-execchoice.co.uk

General Medical Council, 178–202 Great Portland Street, London W1N 6JE. *Tel*: 020 7580 7642.

General Practitioner Writers Association. Membership details from The General Secretary, GPWA, 633 Liverpool Road, Southport, Merseyside PR8 3NG. *Tel*: 01704 577 839; *E-mail*: gpwa@lepress.demon.co.uk

Home Office, Immigration and Nationality Directorate, Lunar House, Wellesley Road, Croydon CR9 2BY. *Tel*: 0870 606 7766.

Institute of Personnel and Development (IPD). Publications and training packs in topics related to career developmement. Distributors: Plymbridge Distributors Ltd, Estover, Plymouth PL6 7PZ. *Internet*: http://www.ipd.co.uk

Joint Committee on Postgraduate Training for General Practice, 14 Princes Gate, Hyde Park, London SW7 1PU. *Tel*: 020 7581 3232.

Media Medics. Dr Paul Stillman, Claybrooke, Haywards, Pound Hill, Crawley, Sussex RH10 3TR. *Tel*: 01293 889100; *Fax*: 01293 882100.

Medical Forum. Offers independent career guidance and personal development for health career professionals, in person, as small group workshops and by e-mail career coaching. Dr Sonia Hutton-Taylor, Director, Greyhound House, 24 George Street, Richmond TW9 1HY. *Internet*: http://fast. to/medicalforum

Medical Officers of Schools Association (MOSA). Issues guideline fee scales. C/o Amherst Medical Practice, 21 St Botolph's Road, Sevenoaks, Kent TN13 3AQ.

Medical Women's Federation. Has careers advisers in each NHS region in England, Wales and Scotland. MWF, BMA House, Tavistock Square, London WC1H 9JP.

National Association of Non-Principals, PO Box 188, Chichester, West Sussex PO19 2ZA. *Fax*: 01243 536428; *Internet*: www.nanp.org.uk

Oxford Psychologists Press Ltd for Myers Briggs instrument and psychological type. Lambourne House, 311–321 Banbury Road, Oxford OX2 7JH. *Tel*: 01865 510203.

Specialist Training Authority, 70 Wimpole Street, London W1M 7DE. *Tel*: 020 7935 8586.

UK Register of Expert Witnesses, c/o Debby Dyson, JS Publications, PO Box 505, Newmarket, Suffolk CB8 7TF.

Women in Medicine. An organisation of women doctors and medical students. Runs local support groups, annual conference, newsletter. 21 Wallingford Avenue, London W10 6QA.

# National sources of help for doctors with stress or mental health problems

National Counselling Service for Sick Doctors. A confidential, independent advisory service for sick doctors, supported by senior doctors in all branches of the profession who act as advisers. *Tel*: 0870 241 0535.

BMA Counselling. A 24-hour confidential telephone counselling service for doctors and their families, and medical students to discuss personal, and work related problems. *Tel*: 0645 200 169.

British Doctors and Dentists Group. For addicted doctors, dentists and their families, giving confidential help and advice. *Tel*: 020 7487 4445.

# Important contact details in your locality

Fill in the details about local career counsellors, or GP, clinical or college tutors or advisers who have specialist knowledge and are willing to see and advise local doctors about career paths.

Your local contacts for careers advice or information:

|  | **Name** | **Contact details** |
|---|---|---|
| **General practice** | | |
| **General surgery** | | |
| **General medicine** | | |
| **Dermatology** | | |

**Public health**

**Paediatrics**

**Anaesthetics**

**Obstetrics and gynaecology**

**Community clinical medical officer**

**Palliative medicine**

**Adviser for flexible training**

**Adviser for career help for poorly performing doctors**

**Adviser for careers of non-principal GPs or non-specialist hospital-based doctors**

**Career counsellors:**
(i)    **non-medical career counsellor**

(ii)   medically trained
        career counsellor

(iii)  **BMA careers
        information: regional office**

(iv)   **local source of
        career counselling or
        advice, e.g. health authority,
        LMC, university**

**Local sources of help
for doctors under
stress, in distress**

**Local sources of help
for doctors with substance
abuse problems**

# INDEX